Clinical Dental Pharmacology

Clinical Dental Pharmacology

Edited by

Kamran Ali

Qatar University
QU Health
College of Dental Medicine
Doha
Qatar

WILEY Blackwell

This edition first published 2024
© 2024 John Wiley & Sons Ltd

All rights reserved. No part of this publication may be reproduced, stored in a retrieval system, or transmitted, in any form or by any means, electronic, mechanical, photocopying, recording or otherwise, except as permitted by law. Advice on how to obtain permission to reuse material from this title is available at http://www.wiley.com/go/permissions.

The right of Kamran Ali to be identified as the author of the editorial material in this work has been asserted in accordance with law.

Registered Offices
John Wiley & Sons, Inc., 111 River Street, Hoboken, NJ 07030, USA
John Wiley & Sons Ltd, The Atrium, Southern Gate, Chichester, West Sussex, PO19 8SQ, UK

For details of our global editorial offices, customer services, and more information about Wiley products visit us at www.wiley.com.

Wiley also publishes its books in a variety of electronic formats and by print-on-demand. Some content that appears in standard print versions of this book may not be available in other formats.

Trademarks: Wiley and the Wiley logo are trademarks or registered trademarks of John Wiley & Sons, Inc. and/or its affiliates in the United States and other countries and may not be used without written permission. All other trademarks are the property of their respective owners. John Wiley & Sons, Inc. is not associated with any product or vendor mentioned in this book.

Limit of Liability/Disclaimer of Warranty
The contents of this work are intended to further general scientific research, understanding, and discussion only and are not intended and should not be relied upon as recommending or promoting scientific method, diagnosis, or treatment by physicians for any particular patient. In view of ongoing research, equipment modifications, changes in governmental regulations, and the constant flow of information relating to the use of medicines, equipment, and devices, the reader is urged to review and evaluate the information provided in the package insert or instructions for each medicine, equipment, or device for, among other things, any changes in the instructions or indication of usage and for added warnings and precautions. While the publisher and authors have used their best efforts in preparing this work, they make no representations or warranties with respect to the accuracy or completeness of the contents of this work and specifically disclaim all warranties, including without limitation any implied warranties of merchantability or fitness for a particular purpose. No warranty may be created or extended by sales representatives, written sales materials or promotional statements for this work. The fact that an organization, website, or product is referred to in this work as a citation and/or potential source of further information does not mean that the publisher and authors endorse the information or services the organization, website, or product may provide or recommendations it may make. This work is sold with the understanding that the publisher is not engaged in rendering professional services. The advice and strategies contained herein may not be suitable for your situation. You should consult with a specialist where appropriate. Further, readers should be aware that websites listed in this work may have changed or disappeared between when this work was written and when it is read. Neither the publisher nor authors shall be liable for any loss of profit or any other commercial damages, including but not limited to special, incidental, consequential, or other damages.

Library of Congress Cataloging-in-Publication Data

Names: Ali, Kamran, editor.
Title: Clinical dental pharmacology / edited by Kamran Ali.
Description: Hoboken, NJ : Wiley-Blackwell, 2024. | Includes index.
Identifiers: LCCN 2024009202 (print) | LCCN 2024009203 (ebook) | ISBN
    9781119984931 (paperback) | ISBN 9781119984948 (Adobe PDF) | ISBN
    9781119984955 (epub)
Subjects: MESH: Pharmaceutical Preparations, Dental–pharmacology | Tooth
    Diseases–drug therapy | Pharmacology, Clinical
Classification: LCC RK305 (print) | LCC RK305 (ebook) | NLM QV 50 | DDC
    617.6/3061–dc23/eng/20240314
LC record available at https://lccn.loc.gov/2024009202
LC ebook record available at https://lccn.loc.gov/2024009203

Cover Design: Wiley
Cover Images: Courtesy of Kamran Ali

Set in 9.5/12pt STIXTwoText by Straive, Chennai, India
Printed and bound by CPI Group (UK) Ltd, Croydon, CR0 4YY

C9781119984931_120424

My late parents for their relentless sacrifices and dedication;
their loving memories continue to inspire me.

My dear wife, Mahwish, for her unwavering support, patience, and understanding.

My beloved sons, Asad and Turab, the greatest blessings in my life.

Contents

List of Contributors

Kamran Ali
Qatar University
QU Health
College of Dental Medicine
Doha
Qatar

Sadeq Ali Al-Maweri
Qatar University
QU Health
College of Dental Medicine
Doha
Qatar

Gail V.A. Douglas
School of Dentistry
University of Leeds
Leeds
UK

Manal Matoug-Elwerfelli
Qatar University
QU Health
College of Dental Medicine
Doha
Qatar

Ewen McColl
Plymouth University
Faculty of Health
(Medicine, Dentistry, and Human Sciences)
Department of Clinical Dentistry
Plymouth
UK

Mahwish Raja
Qatar University
QU Health
College of Dental Medicine
Doha
Qatar

Susu M. Zughaier
Qatar University
QU Health
College of Dental Medicine
Doha
Qatar

Preface

It is a pleasure to share this book entitled *Clinical Dental Pharmacology*. Although there a large number of resources on pharmacology, there has been a long-standing need for a comprehensive text to support decision-making regarding drug prescriptions in clinical dental practice. I am positive that the book will address this gap and serve as an authentic resource for dental professionals and students alike.

The book covers common drugs prescribed by dental practitioners as well as systemic medications which may impact on provision of clinical dental care. A separate section on recognition and management common medical emergencies in dental practice is also included. Pharmacology is a complex subject and a plethora of new information on drugs emerges regularly. Dental professionals may find it difficult to keep pace with latest research and how different drugs may impact on their dental practice. The readers are signposted to professional guidelines from a variety of online sources to facilitate access to evidence-based and reliable information on each topic covered in the book. The readers are advised to consult the guidelines directly from the relevant websites to read the most updated version of the guidelines. Each chapter also includes online resources which can be used for patient education.

The book is aimed at a global audience and covers a wide range of topics. Dental professionals are reminded to consider their scope of practice in the light of national legislation and professional regulations and guidelines applicable to their geographic location. All health professionals must always act in the best interests of the patients and if management of a patient is beyond the expertise of a dental professional, it is best to seek advice from an appropriate colleague or specialist.

I am grateful to all authors for their excellent contributions.

Qatar University
QU Health College of Dental Medicine
Doha, Qatar
08 December 2023

KAMRAN ALI

Abbreviations

A&E	accident and emergency	LA	local anaesthesia
ACE	angiotensin-converting enzyme	LN	lingual nerve
AHA	American Heart Association	LOC	loss of consciousness
b.i.d.	bis in die – twice daily	Mane	in the morning
b.i.d.	quarter in die – four times daily	MAO	mono amino oxidase
BLS	basic life support	mg	milli gram
BNF	British National Formulary	MI	myocardial infarction
BP	blood pressure	mL	milli litre
BT	bleeding time	Nocte	at night
COPD	chronic obstructive pulmonary disease	°C	degree Celsius
		OD	once daily
CPR	cardiopulmonary resuscitation	°F	degree Fahrenheit
CVA	cerebrovascular accident	OSA	obstructive sleep apnoea
DM	diabetes mellitus	OTC	over the counter
DNF	dental national formulary	PO	per oral (by mouth)
EU	European Union	ppm	parts per million
⁻F	fluoride ion	PT	prothrombin time
HHV	human herpes virus	q.i.d.	quater in die – four times daily
HR	heart rate	s.c.	subcutaneous
IAN	inferior alveolar nerve	Stat	statim – immediately
IDN	inferior dental nerve	t.i.d.	ter in die – three times daily
IHD	ischaemic heart disease	TCA	tricyclic antidepressant
IM	intramuscular	tsp	teaspoon
INR	international normalised ratio	U.S.P.	United States pharmacopeia
ION	infra orbital nerve	w	with
IV	intravenous	w/o	without

Medications for Pain Control

Analgesics

CHAPTER 1

Kamran Ali

Qatar University, QU Health, College of Dental Medicine, Doha, Qatar

1.1 INTRODUCTION

One of the commonest presenting complaint of patients in dentistry is pain, and dentists routinely advise/prescribe analgesics. However, the main purpose of analgesics is to provide symptomatic relief before definitive treatment and minimise pain following operative interventions. Pain control during operative dental procedures is usually accomplished with administration of local anaesthesia (Chapter 3). Appropriate management of dental and orofacial pain should address the cause of pain using a comprehensive clinical assessment and relevant investigations such as radiographs. For example, patients presenting with features of pulpitis may benefit from analgesics to achieve pain relief, and definitive pain relief is best obtained through operative management of the inflamed pulp. Similarly, the use of analgesics to manage pain related to a peri-radicular abscess can only provide a partial and temporary relief, at best. Definitive management of the abscess would require drainage of the abscess through root canal access opening or tooth extraction, as appropriate.

Some of the key principles which need to be observed when prescribing analgesics in dentistry are summarised as follows:

- *Undertake a comprehensive clinical assessment*
  Before advising or prescribing an analgesic, it is important to assess the source of pain along with its character, severity, site, frequency, aggravating and relieving factors to aid an accurate diagnosis.

- *Choose an appropriate analgesic*
  The choice of analgesic will depend on the cause and severity of pain as well as the patient's medical history and any contraindications. All medications have potential risks and benefits, and the choice of an analgesic should take into account the patient's systemic health, and any potential drug interactions of the proposed analgesics with any medications the patient may be taking.

- *Determine route of administration*
  In most cases, analgesics used for the management of pain in dental patients are administered orally. However, for pain associated with certain chronic conditions, such as myofascial pain and internal derangement of temporomandibular joint, topical application may be appropriate to minimise the systemic side effects associated with long-term use of oral analgesics. Parenteral administration of analgesics for acute dental pain is usually not undertaken in general dental practice settings. Nevertheless, local anaesthetic administration can be used for immediate management of severe acute pain.

- *Determine the dose and duration of analgesics cover*
  Analgesics should be used at the lowest effective dose for the shortest duration necessary. This can help reduce the risk of side effects and addiction and minimise the cost. In most

Clinical Dental Pharmacology, First Edition. Edited by Kamran Ali.
© 2024 John Wiley & Sons Ltd. Published 2024 by John Wiley & Sons Ltd.

cases analgesics used for the management of acute dental pain are administered orally for few days until definitive management of the underlying problem. Similarly post-operative pain following invasive dental procedures requires analgesics for up to a week. However, pain associated with certain chronic conditions such as temporomandibular joint disorders (e.g., myofascial pain and internal derangement) and trigeminal neuralgia may require long-term analgesics. As mentioned before, topical application of analgesics may be considered if appropriate to minimise the systemic side effects associated with long-term use of analgesics.

- *Consider the cost of analgesics*
  Many analgesics used in dentistry are available over the counter, and it may be much cheaper for the patients to purchase these themselves on a dentist's advice. Dispensing analgesics on a prescription may be more expensive for patients in many countries.

- *Patient education and follow-up*
  Patients should be advised to read the patient information leaflet (PIL), accompanying the medication. The patients should be advised on how to take the medication safely and effectively. Also, precautions, side effects or adverse reactions to the medication and appropriate actions which may be required should be discussed. Patients should be followed up to ensure that the medication is effective and welltolerated and to make any necessary adjustments to the treatment plan.

1.2 NON-NARCOTIC ANALGESICS

Non-narcotic analgesics, also known as non-steroidal anti-inflammatory drugs (NSAIDs), are the most frequently used analgesics across the board in clinical medicine as well as dentistry. In addition to their analgesic effects, these drugs also have anti-inflammatory, antipyretic and antiplatelet activity. These drugs are widely used for short-term management of mild to moderate pain from various causes including dental pain. More severe pain, particularly of visceral origin, may require management with opioid analgesics either alone or in combination with NSAIDs.

1.2.1 MECHANISM OF ACTION

Tissue injury leads to breakdown of membrane phospholipids by the enzyme phospholipase A_2 (PLA_2). This results in the release of arachidonic acid (AA) from the membrane phospholipids. AA is metabolised via the cyclooxygenase (COX) and lipoxygenase (LOX) pathways as depicted in Figure 1.1.

Most NSAIDs are non-selective inhibitors of COX and target the two main isoforms of COX, i.e., COX-1 and COX-2. COX catalyses the formation of prostaglandins and thromboxane from AA. Aspirin inhibits COX irreversibly, while the other NSAIDs (e.g., indomethacin and diclofenac) cause reversible inhibition of COX. Steroids inhibit PLA_2 and block both the COX and LOX pathways.

The analgesic effect results from inhibition of prostaglandin synthesis (especially inhibition of PGE_2) as well as inhibition of bradykinin release from high-molecular-weight (HMW) kininogens in the blood plasma and tissues.

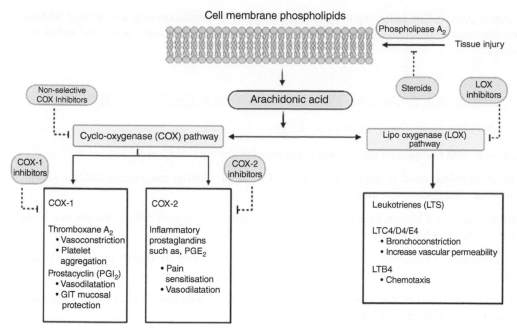

FIGURE 1.1 Mechanism of action of non-steroidal anti-inflammatory drugs. Source: Image created in BioRender.com

1.2.2 SIDE EFFECTS

The main side effects of NSAIDs are gastric imitation, nephrotoxicity and hypersensitivity (also see individual drugs).

1.2.3 SELECTIVE COX-2 INHIBITORS

Traditional NSAIDs, such as aspirin, ibuprofen and naproxen, block both isoforms of COX, i.e., COX-1 and COX-2, which can lead to unwanted side effects such as stomach ulcers and bleeding.

COX-2 inhibitors are a class of drugs that selectively block the enzyme cyclooxygenase-2 (COX-2). The rationale for using COX-2 inhibitors is to reduce inflammation and pain without affecting the other functions of COX-1, another form of the enzyme that is involved in the production of protective prostaglandins that help maintain the health of the stomach lining and regulate blood clotting.

However, COX-2 inhibitors have been associated with an increased risk of cardiovascular events such as heart attack and stroke, particularly when used at high doses or for long periods of time. This has led to a sharp decline in the use of COX-2 inhibitors. Although some COX-2 inhibitors (e.g., celecoxib and meloxicam) may still be used for short-term pain relief associated with conditions such as osteoarthritis, and rheumatoid arthritis, there is little indication for their use in dentistry. Extreme caution is required when using COX-2 inhibitors in patients with cardiovascular risk factors and medical advice must be sought.

NSAIDs are used as first-line therapy for acute dental pain. Paracetamol and ibuprofen alone or in combination are one of the most common NSAIDs used in the management of oral surgical and dental pain[1-3]. The following section discusses the most common oral and topical NSAIDS which are used in the management of pain and inflammation associated with oral and dental disorders.

1.3 COMMON NON-STEROIDAL ANTI-INFLAMMATORY AGENTS USED IN DENTISTRY

1.3.1 ASPIRIN (ACETYL SALICYLIC ACID)

Indications: Mild to moderate pain, pyrexia, antiplatelet activity (see Chapter 15).

Cautions: Impaired renal or hepatic function; dehydration; elderly; pregnancy; asthma, allergic disease; alcohol (gastric bleeding).

Contra-indications: Children under 12 years, breastfeeding, gastrointestinal ulceration, and blood dyscrasias such as haemophilia and thrombocytopenia.

Hypersensitivity: Contraindicated in patients with hypersensitivity to aspirin or other NSAIDs; asthma; angioedema; rhinitis; urticaria.

Side effects: GIT irritation; slight asymptomatic blood loss; increased bleeding time; bronchospasm; skin reactions in hypersensitive patients.

Interactions: Enhances effects or oral anticoagulants (bleeding); oral hypoglycaemics (hypogly-caemia); corticosteroids (peptic ulceration).

***COMMERCIAL PREPARATIONS*:**
Aspirin
  Tablets, aspirin 300 mg

***ROUTE OF ADMINISTRATION AND DOSE*:**
By mouth, 300–900 mg every 4–6 hours, maximum 4 g daily. Child not recommended.

1.3.2 PARACETAMOL (ACETAMINOPHEN)

Paracetamol is one of the most widely used analgesic and antipyretic worldwide. It is similar to aspirin in efficacy but has no demonstrable anti-inflammatory/antiplatelet activity; it is less irritant to the stomach than aspirin, and thus it is generally preferred to aspirin, especially in the elderly.

Indications: Mild to moderate pain, pyrexia.

Cautions: Hepatic and renal impairment; alcohol dependence.

Side effects: Rashes; blood disorders; acute pancreatitis reported after prolonged use; liver damage; renal damage (less frequently).

Overdosage: Nausea, vomiting, right subcostal pain; hepatocellular necrosis; renal necrosis.

***COMMERCIAL PREPARATIONS*:**

Panadol®

  Soluble tablets, paracetamol 500 mg
  Oral suspension, paracetamol 250 mg/5 mL
  Oral suspension, paracetamol 120 mg/5 mL

***ROUTE OF ADMISSION AND DOSE*:**

By mouth, 0.5 g every 4–6 hours, maximum 4 g daily. Child 1–5 years 120–250 mg and 6–12 years 250–500 mg.

1.3.3 IBUPROFEN

Indications: Fever; pain and inflammation; mild to moderate pain; post-operative analgesia; musculoskeletal disorders including pain related to the temporomandibular joint.

Cautions: Hypersensitivity to other NSAIDs; asthma, Crohn's disease, ulcerative colitis; over 65 years.

Contra-indications: Renal impairment; cardiac impairment; hepatic impairment; peptic ulceration.

Side effects: GIT discomfort, nausea, diarrhoea, bleeding, ulceration occasionally; hypersensitivity reactions; headache, dizziness; vertigo.

***COMMERCIAL PREPARATIONS AND DOSE*:**
Nurofen®
  Caplets, ibuprofen, 200 mg
  Liquid capsules, ibuprofen 400 mg
  Caplets, ibuprofen, 684 mg
  Dose: 1.2–1.8 g daily in 3–4 divided doses, maximum 2.4 g daily.
  Paediatric:
  Chewable capsules, ibuprofen 100 mg
  Oral suspension, ibuprofen 100 mg/5 mL
  Dose: 20 mg/kg daily.

Brufen®
  Coated tablets, ibuprofen 200 mg, 400 mg, 600 mg
  Syrup, 100 mg/5 mL
  Granules effervescent, 600 mg/sachet
  Dose: 1.2–1.8 g daily in 3–4 divided doses, maximum 2.4 g daily; child 20mg/kg daily not for children under 7 years.

Brufen Retard®
  Tablets, m/r, ibuprofen 800 mg
  Dose: 2 tablets daily as a single dose, preferably in the early evening, increased in severe cases to 3 tablets in 2 divided doses. Child not recommended.

Topical
  Ibugel®
  Topical, ibuprofen gel 5%; apply 3 times daily.

1.3.4 NAPROXEN

Indications: Similar to ibuprofen.

Cautions: *Contra-indications*: *Side effects*: Similar to ibuprofen, though slightly more.

COMMERCIAL PREPARATIONS AND DOSE:
Naprosyn®
  Tablets, naproxen 250 mg, 375 mg, 500 mg; available as gastro-resistant enteric-coated preparations
  Dose: 500 mg twice daily, preferably after food. Child under 16 years not recommended.

Synflex®
  Tablets, naproxen sodium 550 mg
  Dose: 500 mg twice daily, preferably after food. Child under 16 years not recommended.

1.3.5 FLURBIPROFEN

Indications: Similar to ibuprofen.

Cautions: *Contra-indications*: *Side effects*: Similar to ibuprofen, though slightly more.

COMMERCIAL PREPARATIONS AND DOSE:
Froben®
  Tablets, flurbiprofen 50 mg
  Dose: By mouth, 150–200 mg daily divided doses, increased in acute conditions to 300 mg daily. Child not recommended.

Froben SR®
  Capsules, m/r, flurbiprofen 200 mg
  Dose: 1 capsule daily, preferably in the evening. Child not recommended.

Ansaid®
  Tablets, flurbiprofen 100 mg
  Dose: By mouth, 150–200 mg daily divided doses, increased in acute conditions to 300 mg daily. Child not recommended.

1.3.6 MEFENAMIC ACID

Indications: Similar to ibuprofen.

Cautions: *Contra-indications*: Similar to other NSAIDs; especially contraindicated in inflammatory bowel disease; blood tests required during long-term treatment; porphyria.

Interactions: Enhances effects of oral anticoagulants (bleeding); oral hypoglycaemics (hypoglycaemia).

Side effects: Drowsiness; diarrhoea or rashes (withdraw treatment); thrombocytopenia, haemolyticanaemia and aplastic anaemia; convulsions on overdose.

COMMERCIAL PREPARATIONS:
Ponstan®
  Capsules, mefenamic acid 250 mg
  Paediatric oral suspension, mefenamic acid 50 mg/5 mL

Ponstan Forte®
  Tablets, mefenamic acid 500 mg

ROUTE OF ADMINISTRATION AND DOSE:
By mouth, 500 mg 3 times daily preferably after food. Child over 6 months, 25 mg/kg daily in divided doses for not longer than 7 days, except in juvenile arthritis.

1.3.7 DICLOFENAC SODIUM

Indications: Similar to ibuprofen.

Cautions: *Contra-indications*: *Side effects*: Similar to naproxen (see earlier notes); avoid in porphyria.

COMMERCIAL PREPARATIONS AND DOSE:
Voltarol®
  Tablets e/c diclofenac sodium, 25 mg, 50 mg
  Dose: By mouth, 75–150 mg daily in 2–3 divided doses, preferably after food.
  Maximum total daily dose by any route 150 mg.

Voltarol 75 mg SR®
  Tablets m/r diclofenac sodium, 75 mg
  Dose: By mouth, 75 mg 1–2 times daily, preferably with food. Child not recommended.

Topical
  Emulgel®
    Diclofenac dimethylammonium salt, 1.16% (equivalent to diclofenac sodium 1%). Apply 3–4 times daily.

1.3.8 INDOMETHACIN

Indications: Mild to moderate pain and inflammation; musculoskeletal disorders including temporomandibular joint.

Cautions: *Contra-indications*: Caution in epilepsy, parkinsonism psychiatric disturbances; blood and ophthalmic examination are advised during prolonged therapy; avoid rectal administration in proctitis and haemorrhoids. Dizziness may affect the performance of skilled tasks, e.g., driving.

Side effects: Similar to naproxen (see earlier notes); frequently GIT disturbances (including diarrhoea) GIT ulceration and bleeding headache, dizziness, light-headedness; rarely confusion, insomnia, convulsions, depression, syncope; blood disorders (particularly thrombocytopenia), hypertension, hyperglycaemia, blurred vision, and peripheral neuropathy.

COMMERCIAL PREPARATIONS AND DOSE:
Indocid®
  Capsules, indomethacin 25 mg, 50 mg
  Suspension, indomethacin 25 mg/5 mL
  Dose: By mouth, 50–200 mg daily in divided doses with food. Child not recommended.
  Maximum total daily dose by any route 150–200 mg.

Indocid R®
  Capsules, m/r indomethacin 75 mg
  Dose: By mouth, 75 mg 1–2 times daily preferably with food. Child not recommended.

1.4 NARCOTIC ANALGESICS

Narcotic analgesics, also known as opioids, are a class of strong pain-relieving medications that are derived from the opium poppy plant or synthesised to mimic the effects of these natural substances. Narcotic analgesics work by binding to opioid receptors in the brain and spinal cord, which can result in pain relief, sedation, and euphoria.

Opioid overdose is a growing public health problem globally and has given rise to an opioid crisis in the United States and Canada with an estimated 600,000 deaths due to opioid overdose in the last two decades[4]. Opioid prescriptions have also increased in the United Kingdom and have been associated with a remarkable increase in incidences of overdose and hospitalisations[5]. Like other health professionals, dentists should also limit the use of narcotic analgesics due to risks of addiction and overdose. Narcotic analgesics should be prescribed when absolutely necessary, and the dose should be kept low and the duration must also be limited.

1.4.1 MECHANISM OF ACTION

Opioids combine selectively with many recognition sites throughout the body. Brain loci involved in the transmission of pain and in the alteration of reactivity to nociceptive (painful) stimuli appear to be primary site of opioid action. Specific opioid receptors (Mu, kappa, sigma, and delta receptors) are distributed in the dorsal horn of spinal cord, certain subcortical regions of the brain, and also in several thalamic and hypothalamic areas – the major areas of central nervous system (CNS) concerned with nociception. These nociceptive sites in the brain also contain high concentrations of endogenous peptides (opiopeptins) such as β-endorphin and enkephalins which have opiate-like properties. These endogenous peptides are released from the brain as a physiological response to pain. Morphine and other opioid analgesics mimic the action of these endogenous ligands with their receptors; this interaction gives rise to their pharmacological effects.

Neurotransmitters showing depressed release after opioid administration include acetylcholine, norepinephrine, dopamine, 5-hydroxytryptamine and substance P. This depressed release of neurotransmitters is related to decreased calcium entry or enhanced potassium entry across specific ion channels. However, chronic exposure to opioids leads to an elevation of intracellular calcium; this mechanism is responsible for tolerance and physical dependence.

1.4.2 SIDE EFFECTS

Opioid analgesics share many side effects, though qualitative and quantitative differences exist. The most common include nausea, vomiting, constipation and drowsiness. Larger doses produce respiratory depression and hypotension. Drowsiness may affect the performance of skilled tasks (e.g., driving); effects of alcohol are enhanced. Drug tolerance and dependence is a recognised risk with all narcotic drugs.

1.4.3 OVERDOSE

Varying degrees of coma, respiratory depression, pinpoint pupils (miosis).

Acute opioid overdose may be managed with appropriate antidotes such as naloxone (Narcan®) and Levallorphan (Larfan®).

1.4.4 COMMON NARCOTIC ANALGESICS

A variety of narcotic analgesics are available for medical use including the following:

- Morphine (Oramorph®)
- Diamorphine hydrochloride (Heroin)
- Pethidine (CD Pethidine®)
- Codeine (Codeine phosphate®)

- Fentanyl (Actiq®, Abstral®)

- Oxycodone (Oxaydo®)

- Hydrocodone (Hysingla®)

- Tramadol (Ultram®)

- Buprenorphine (Temgesic®)

Majority of the aforementioned narcotic analgesics are unsuitable in dental settings due to serious side effects and risks associated with their use and are best prescribed under medical care. However, narcotic analgesics mentioned in the following text may be used for the management of pain by dentists.

Codeine Phosphate

Indications: Mild to moderate pain.

Cautions: Hypotension, hypothyroidism, asthma, decreased respiratory reserve, prostatic hypertrophy, pregnancy, breastfeeding; precipitate coma in hepatic impairment, renal impairment; elderly and debilitated; should be avoided altogether in Children less than 1 year.

Contra-indications: Acute respiratory depression; acute alcoholism; paralytic ileus, acute abdomen, raised intracranial pressure, head injury; pheochromocytoma (risk of presser response to histamine release).

Side effects: Nausea, vomiting (initial stages), constipation; drowsiness; larger doses produce respiratory depression, and hypotension, also ureteric or biliary spasm, dry mouth, sweating, headache, flushing, vertigo, bradycardia, tachycardia, palpitations, hypothermia, hallucinations, dysphoria, mood changes, dependence, miosis, decreased libido, rashes, urticaria and pruritus.

Overdosage: Coma, respiratory depression, pinpoint pupils (miosis).

COMMERCIAL PREPARATIONS:
Codeine phosphate®
  Tablets, codeine sulphate 15 mg, 30 mg, 60 mg
  Syrup, codeine sulphate 25 mg/mL

ROUTE OF ADMINISTRATION AND DOSE:
By mouth, 30–60 mg every 4 hours, maximum 240 mg daily. Child 1–12 years, 3 mg/kg daily in divided doses.

COMPOUND PREPARATIONS:
Compound preparations contain a combination of NSAIDs and narcotic analgesics and may be used for management of pain in dental settings.

- *Co-Codamol (Codeine phosphate and paracetamol)*
  Panadeine®
    Tablets, co-codamol 8/500 (codeine phosphate 8 mg, paracetamol 500 mg).
    Dose: 1–2 tablets every 4–6 hours; maximum 8 tablets daily. Child ½–1 tablet.

- *Co-dydramol (dihydrocodeine tartrate and paracetamol)*
  Paramol®
    Tablets, co-dydramol 10/500 (dihydrocodeine tartrate 10 mg, paracetamol 500 mg).
    Dose: 1–2 tablets every 4–6 hours; maximum 8 tablets daily. Child not recommended.

Remedeine®
Tablets, dihydrocodeine tartrate 20 mg, paracetamol 500 mg.
Dose: 1–2 tablets every 4–6 hours; maximum 8 tablets daily. Child not recommended.

- *Codafen (acetaminophen and codeine phosphate)*
Codafein®
Tablets, acetaminophen 300 mg, codeine phosphate 15 mg, caffeine 15 mg.
Dose: 1–2 tablets every 12 hours; maximum 3 tablets every 12 hours. Child not recommended.

RESOURCES

RESOURCES FOR DENTAL PROFESSIONALS

ADA (American Dental Association). Oral analgesics for acute dental pain. https://www.ada.org/resources/research/science-and-research-institute/oral-health-topics/oral-analgesics-for-acute-dental-pain (accessed 25 February 2024).

RESOURCES FOR DENTAL PATIENTS

Mayo Clinic. First aid for Toothache. https://www.mayoclinic.org/first-aid/first-aid-toothache/basics/art-20056628 (accessed 21 March 2024).

Cleveland Clinic. Toothache. https://my.clevelandclinic.org/health/diseases/10957-toothache (accessed 25 February 2024).

REFERENCES

1. Smith, E.A., Marshall, J.G., Selph, S.S. et al. (2017). Nonsteroidal anti-inflammatory drugs for managing postoperative endodontic pain in patients who present with preoperative pain: a systematic review and meta-analysis. *Journal of Endodontics* 43: 7–15.

2. Gately, F., Ali, K., and Burns, L. (2022). The effect of pre-emptive ibuprofen on post-operative pain after removal of lower third molar teeth: a systematic review. *Evidence-Based Dentistry* https://doi.org/10.1038/s41432-021-0211-1.

3. Santini, M.F., da Rosa, R.A., Ferreira, M.B.C. et al. (2021). Medications used for prevention and treatment of postoperative endodontic pain: a systematic review. *European Endodontic Journal* 6: 15.

4. The Lancet Public Health (2022). Opioid overdose crisis: time for a radical rethink. *The Lancet Public Health* 7: e195.

5. Friebel, R. and Maynou, L. (2022). Trends and characteristics of hospitalisations from the harmful use of opioids in England between 2008 and 2018: population-based retrospective cohort study. *Journal of the Royal Society of Medicine* 115 (5): 173–185.

Anti-Neuralgic Medications

CHAPTER 2

Kamran Ali

Qatar University, QU Health, College of Dental Medicine, Doha, Qatar

2.1 INTRODUCTION

Pain in the orofacial region is one of the most common presenting complaints of patients in dental practice. Whilst most cases of pain are related to odontogenic causes, it is not unusual to encounter patients with pain from non-odontogenic causes. Table 2.1 summarises recognised causes of odontogenic and non-odontogenic pain including neuralgias, vascular disorders, psychogenic disorders, drugs, and referred pain[1]. Dentists are expected to be competent in managing odontogenic pain and should also be able to recognise the presentation of pain from a variety of non-odontogenic causes. It is important that patients with non-odontogenic pain are referred to appropriate specialists for definitive management.

2.1.1 GENERAL PRINCIPLES OF MANAGEMENT OF OROFACIAL PAIN

- Pain in the orofacial region is most commonly related to odontogenic causes and other local sources such as the jaw bones, temporomandibular joint, maxillary sinus, and salivary glands.
- Never extract teeth without a definitive diagnosis and justification.
- Always exclude organic cause before labelling the pain as psychogenic.
- Patients with psychogenic disease are not exempt from organic disease.
- Refer to specialists if a definitive diagnosis cannot be established.

2.2 OROFACIAL NEURALGIAS

The term neuralgia refers to pain originating in a nerve pathway and most commonly results from irritation or damage to a nerve or one of its branches. The most common type of neuralgia in the orofacial region is trigeminal neuralgia. Vago-glossopharyngeal neuralgia is also recognised but occurs less frequently. This chapter discusses the medical management of common types of neuralgic pain in the orofacial region.

2.2.1 TRIGEMINAL NEURALGIA

Trigeminal neuralgia involves the distribution of the trigeminal nerve and is the most recognised neuralgia in the orofacial region[2]. Although most cases are idiopathic, the condition may be related to central vascular compression of trigeminal nerve. It is usually seen in the fifth decade or later with a male predilection. The clinical presentation of trigeminal neuralgia is characterised by intense paroxysmal electric or shooting pain unilaterally and any branch of the nerve may be involved. Each bout of pain may last for a few seconds to minutes. Pain is often initiated by touching an area on the face often referred to as a *trigger* zone. The pain may be so severe that

Clinical Dental Pharmacology, First Edition. Edited by Kamran Ali.
© 2024 John Wiley & Sons Ltd. Published 2024 by John Wiley & Sons Ltd.

Table 2.1 Differential Diagnosis of Orofacial Pain

Source of pain	Common disorders
Teeth	Dentin sensitivity
	Pulpitis
	Infected periapical lesions
	Periapical granuloma
	Periapical abscess
	Radicular cyst
Periodontium	Periodontal abscess
	Pericoronitis
	Necrotising periodontal diseases
	HIV-associated periodontal disease
Temporomandibular joint	Arthritis
	Facial arthromyalgia, including myofascial pain and internal derangement of temporomandibular joint (TMJ)
Jaws	Alveolar osteitis (dry socket)
	Fractures
	Osteomyelitis
	Osteoradionecrosis
	Medication-related osteonecrosis of jaws (MRONJ)
	Infected cysts and malignant neoplasms
Maxillary antrum	Acute sinusitis
	Malignant neoplasms
Salivary glands	Acute sialadenitis
	Ductal obstruction
	Malignant neoplasms
	Advanced Sjogren's syndrome
	HIV-associated salivary gland disease
Nerves	*Primary neuralgias*
	Trigeminal neuralgia
	Vago-glossopharyngeal neuralgia
	Secondary neuralgias
	Post-herpetic neuralgia
	Multiple sclerosis neuralgia
	Causalgia
	Neuralgia-inducing cavitational osteonecrosis.
	Intracranial and extracranial mass lesions, e.g., tumours and cysts
	Extracranial mass lesions
	Nasopharyngeal carcinoma (Totter's syndrome)
	HIV-associated neurologic disease
Blood vessels	Migraine
	Cluster headaches
	Temporal arteritis
Psychogenic	Atypical facial pain
	Atypical odontalgia
	Oral dysesthesia
	Facial arthromyalgia
	Factitious ulceration
Referred	Ischemic heart disease (angina pectoris and myocardial infarction)
	Nasopharyngeal, ocular and aural disease

patients may avoid washing their face or shaving. However, it does not usually wake the patient from sleep. The pain does not respond to routine analgesics.

Trigeminal neuralgia may also develop secondary to multiple sclerosis, an immunologically mediated demyelinating nerve disease. Approximately 2–4% of patients presenting with trigeminal neuralgia may have multiple sclerosis and should be ruled out, especially in young adults in the first or second decade.

Diagnosisis based on history, clinical examination, local radiographs and more sophisticated investigations like computerised tomography (CT) scan (to rule out central mass lesions) and MRI (to rule out central vascular compression).

Medical management is usually the first line of treatment[3]. A variety of drugs (discussed later in this chapter) are used in the medical management of trigeminal neuralgia[4]. Operative options include microvascular decompression (MVD), gamma knife radio surgery (GKR) and percutaneous stereotactic radiofrequency thermal rhizotomy (PSRTR). Historically, partial sensory rhizotomy (PSR), glycerol injections, alcohol injections and cryotherapy have also been tried with variable success but are not used in contemporary clinical practice.

2.2.2 MEDICAL MANAGEMENT OF TRIGEMINAL NEURALGIA

There are a wide range of medications which may be effective in the management of trigeminal neuralgia. If dentists in general practice settings encounter patients with suspected trigeminal neuralgia, emergency pain relief may be achieved with one of the common medications described, preferably carbamazepine. However, patients should be referred to specialists in oral medicine, and neurology for an accurate diagnosis and further management.

Carbamazepine

Carbamazepine is the most widely used medication for managing trigeminal neuralgia and remains a first-line treatment option. It is a tricyclic compound chemically related to tricyclic antidepressants (TCAs) with anticonvulsant and analgesic properties. When taken during the acute stages of trigeminal neuralgia, it reduces the frequency and severity of attacks.

Mechanism of action: It is a membrane-stabilising agent and blocks sodium channels at therapeutic concentrations, inhibiting repetitive firing in neurons. It also acts presynaptically to decrease synaptic transmission. These effects account for the anticonvulsant action of carbamazepine. However, these effects are independent of gamma aminobutyric acid (GABA) - an inhibitory neurotransmitter.

Indications: Trigeminal neuralgia; all forms of epilepsy except primary generalised epilepsy and absence seizures; prophylaxis in manic-depressive illness.

Cautions: Hepatic or renal impairment; cardiac disease, skin reactions; history of haematological reactions to other drugs; glaucoma; pregnancy; breastfeeding; avoid sudden withdrawal.

Contraindications: AV conduction abnormalities (unless paced); history of bone marrow depression, porphyria.

Side effects: Nausea, vomiting, dizziness, headache, ataxia, confusion, and agitation; visual disturbances (especially double vision); constipation or diarrhoea, anorexia; mild generalised transient erythematous rash; leukopenia and other blood disorders (e.g., thrombocytopenia, agranulocytosis, aplastic anaemia); also cholestatic jaundice, hepatitis and acute renal failure; cardiac conduction abnormalities, dyskinesis, paraesthesia, depression, impotence, galactorrhoea, gynecomastia, aggression, activation of psychosis.

Toxicity: Diplopia, ataxia-most common.

Counselling: Blood, hepatic or skin disorders (with all of the above preparations).

Baseline and 6-month full blood counts and liver function tests are advised to monitor side effects of carbamazepine.

COMMERCIAL PREPARATIONS:

Tegretol®

Tablets, carbamazepine 100 mg, 200 mg, 400 mg
Chew tabs, carbamazepine 100 mg, 200 mg, 400 mg
Liquid, carbamazepine 100 mg/5 mL, 200 mg, 400 mg
Suppositories, carbamazepine 125 mg, 250 mg, 400 mg

Tegretol Retard®

Tablets, m/r, carbamazepine 200 mg, 400 mg

ROUTE OF ADMINISTRATION AND DOSE:

By mouth, initially 100 mg once or twice daily and increased slowly until the best response is obtained; most patients require 200 mg 3–4 times daily; maximum daily is 1600 g (in divided doses). Plasma concentrations of the drug should be determined with higher doses. Optimal therapeutic plasma concentration of carbamazepine ranges from 4 to 12 mg/L.

Oxcarbazepine

Structurally similar to carbamazepine, oxcarbazepine may be tolerated by patients better due to fewer side effects.

Mechanism of action: Like carbamazepine, oxcarbazepine binds to sodium channels and inhibits high-frequency repetitive neuronal firing.

Indications: Trigeminal neuralgia; epilepsy.

Cautions: Hepatic impairment; skin reactions; history of haematological reactions to other drugs; breastfeeding; avoid sudden withdrawal.

Side effects: Nausea, vomiting, abdominal pain, sedation, dizziness, headache, ataxia, fatigue, confusion, or rashes, diplopia, liver damage.

Contra-indications: Myoclonus, pregnancy, hypersensitivity.

COMMERCIAL PREPARATIONS:

Trileptal®

Tablets, oxcarbazepine 150 mg, 300 mg, 600 mg
Oral suspension, oxcarbazepine 300 mg/5 mL

Oxtellar XR®

Tablets, oxcarbazepine extended release 150 mg, 300 mg, 600 mg
Oral suspension, oxcarbazepine 300 mg/5 mL

ROUTE OF ADMINISTRATION AND DOSE:

By mouth, initially 300 mg 8–12 hourly on an empty stomach, and increased slowly until the best response is obtained, up to a 200 mg in divided doses.

Gabapentin

Gabapentin is a structural analogue of anticonvulsant drug γ-aminobutyric acid and is used as a second line of management in trigeminal neuralgia[5].

Mechanism of action: The precise mechanism through which gabapentin exerts its therapeutic effects is unclear. The most widely accepted mode of action is inhibition of voltage-gated calcium channels and subsequent release of excitatory neurotransmitters.

Indications: Neuropathic pain, diabetic neuropathy and seizure disorders.

Cautions: Potentiates the effects of alcohol and other central nervous system (CNS) depressants; may affect vision and ability to drive.

Contraindications: Myasthenia gravis.

Side effects: Nausea, vomiting tiredness, dizziness. Headache, speech difficulties, memory loss, mood changes, depression, tremors, jerky movements, unusual eye movements, blurred vision, diplopia, weight gain.

COMMERCIAL PREPARATIONS:

Neurontin®

Tablets, gabapentin 100 mg, 300 mg, 400 mg
Capsules, gabapentin 300 mg, 600 mg, 800 mg
Oral solution 250 mg/5 mL

ROUTE OF ADMINISTRATION AND DOSE:

By mouth, initial dose of 100–300 mg daily; may be increased to 2400 mg in divided doses.

Phenytoin

Phenytoin may be beneficial in some case of trigeminal neuralgia. It can be given alone or in conjunction with carbamazepine. A combination of phenytoin and carbamazepine is only required in refractory cases or in those with intolerable to high doses of carbamazepine.

Mechanism of action: The mechanism of action of phenytoin involves a combination of actions at several levels; the major action being to block sodium channels at therapeutic concentrations, and inhibiting generation of repetitive action potentials.

Indications: Trigeminal neuralgia; all forms of epilepsy except absence seizures.

Cautions: Hepatic impairment; skin reactions; history of haematological reactions to other drugs; breastfeeding; avoid sudden withdrawal.

Side effects: Nausea, vomiting, dizziness, headache, mental confusion, transient nervousness, insomnia, tremors; gingival hyperplasia, and tenderness; rarely ataxia, dyskinesis, peripheral neuropathy; slurred speech nystagmus and blurred vision; rash epidermal necrolysis, erythema multiforme, lymphadenopathy; hirsutism, acne; leukopenia and other blood disorders, e.g., thrombocytopenia, agranulocytosis, megaloblastic anaemia; also plasma calcium may be lowered (rickets and osteomalacia); hepatitis.

COMMERCIAL PREPARATIONS:

Epanutin®

Capsules, phenytoin sodium 50 mg, 100 mg, 400 mg
Infatabs (= tablets, chewable) phenytoin sodium 50 mg
Suspension, phenytoin 30 mg/5 mL

ROUTE OF ADMINISTRATION AND DOSE:

By mouth, initially 3–4 mg/kg (150–300 mg) daily as a single dose or in 2 divided doses, and increased slowly until the best response is obtained, take after food; most patients require 300–400 mg daily, maximum 600 mg daily; Child, daily in 1–2 divided doses, 5–8 mg/kg. Plasma concentrations of the drug should be determined with higher doses. The optimal plasma concentration for phenytoin is 10–20 mg/mL.

Other medications which may be used in the management of trigeminal neuralgia, primarily in specialist settings, include the following:

- *Skeletal muscle relaxants*: Baclofen
- *Tricyclic antidepressants*: Amitriptyline, Nortriptyline
- *Anticonvulsants*: Pregabalin, Valproic acid, Clonazepam, Lamotrigine, Topiramate
- Opioids.

2.2.3 VAGO-GLOSSOPHARYNGEAL NEURALGIA

Vago-glossopharyngeal neuralgia is a rare type of primary neuralgia affecting the vagus and glossopharyngeal nerve. It is approximately 100 times less common than trigeminal neuralgia. Presentation is similar to trigeminal neuralgia except for the location of pain which is often localised to the base of tongue, pharynx and tonsillar areas and may also involve the ear and infra-auricular areas. Management principles are generally similar to those for trigeminal neuralgia. If identified in general dental practice settings, patients with vago-glossopharyngeal neuralgia may be referred to specialists in oral medicine, ENT or neurology.

2.2.4 POST-HERPETIC NEURALGIA

Post-herpetic neuralgia (PHN) is an extremely painful condition that develops as a complication of infection with human herpes virus (HHV) type 3. Primary infection with HHV-3 causes chicken pox, while reactivation of HHV-3 manifests as herpes zoster or shingles (see Chapter 8). Although most cases of herpes zoster resolve in 2–4 weeks, the herpes zoster virus infection may cause persistent inflammation and damage to nerve fibres leading to altered pain signalling and persistent pain after the skin lesions associated with herpes zoster have healed. Pain lasting for over a month after herpes zoster infection is termed post-herpetic neuralgia.

Clinically, PHN presents with persistent, severe and debilitating pain and is usually localised to the site of skin lesions of shingles. Patients may also experience hypersensitivity, such as burning, itching, or sharp, stabbing pains. PHN can significantly impact a person's daily activities, sleep and overall quality of life.

Diagnosis of PHN is primarily based on clinical grounds as the patient's history of shingles and the presence of persistent pain in the affected area after the rash has healed is adequate for its diagnosis.

Management of PHN include the use of topical anaesthetics such as lidocaine gel or skin patches (see Chapter 3) to alleviate localised pain. Systemic medications used in the management of PHN include oral anticonvulsants (Gabapentin), TCAs (amitriptyline or nortriptyline) and opioids (in severe cases). Opioids should be used cautiously due to the risk of dependence and other side effects (see Chapter 1). Other options include transcutaneous electrical nerve stimulation (TENS), and acupuncture along with counselling, cognitive behavioural therapy may also be beneficial.

Prevention of shingles may be achieved through vaccination (see Chapter 8).

RESOURCES

RESOURCES FOR DENTAL PROFESSIONALS

The American Association of Neurological Surgeons. Trigeminal neuralgia. https://www.aans
.org/Patients/Neurosurgical-Conditions-and-Treatments/Trigeminal-Neuralgia (accessed 28
February 2024).

RESOURCES FOR DENTAL PATIENTS

Mayo Clinic. Trigeminal neuralgia. https://www.aans.org/Patients/Neurosurgical-Conditions-
and-Treatments/Trigeminal-Neuralgia (accessed 25 February 2024).

Cleveland Clinic. Trigeminal neuralgia (TN). https://my.clevelandclinic.org/health/diseases/
15671-trigeminal-neuralgia-tn (accessed 25 February 2024).

REFERENCES

1. Zakrzewska, J.M. (2013). Differential diagnosis of facial pain and guidelines for management. *British Journal of Anaesthesia* 111 (1): 95–104.

2. Van Kleef, M., Van Genderen, W.E., Narouze, S. et al. (2009). Chapter 1: Trigeminal neuralgia. In: *Evidence-Based Interventional Pain Medicine: According to Clinical Diagnoses*, vol. 9 (ed. J. van Zundert, J. Patijn, C.T. Hartrick, et al.), 664–675. Pain Practice.

3. Peterson-Houle, G.M., Abdel Fattah, M.R., Padilla, M., and Enciso, R. (2021). Efficacy of medications in adult patients with trigeminal neuralgia compared to placebo intervention: a systematic review with meta-analyses. *Journal of Dental Anesthesia and Pain Medicine* 21 (5): 379.

4. Cruccu, G., Gronseth, G., Alksne, J. et al. (2008). AAN-EFNS guidelines on trigeminal neuralgia management. *European Journal of Neurology* 15: 1013–1028.

5. Cheshire, W.P. (2002). Defining the role for gabapentin in the treatment of trigeminal neuralgia: a retrospective study. *The Journal of Pain* 3 (2): 137–142.

CHAPTER 3

Local Anaesthetics

Kamran Ali

Qatar University, QU Health, College of Dental Medicine, Doha, Qatar

3.1 INTRODUCTION

Local anaesthetics are the most commonly administered drugs in clinical dentistry and provide the mainstay of pain control during invasive dental procedures. Safe and effective administration of local anaesthesia (LA) is a core skill for dentists and requires a thorough knowledge of regional anatomy, applied pharmacology, skills in the safe assembly of LA equipment and administration of LA using appropriate techniques.

Most routine dental procedures in the maxilla can be accomplished with supra-periosteal infiltration as the maxillary bone is porous and anaesthetic drugs are able to diffuse through the bone to anesthetise the terminal branches of the nerve(s) supplying the operative site. Infiltration is also effective for dental procedures in the anterior mandible. The bone in the posterior mandible (molar and premolar region) is thick, and most dentists administer an inferior alveolar nerve (IAN) block for adequate pain control during invasive dental procedures such as endodontics and tooth extractions. However, an IAN block requires more technical skills and experience compared to an infiltration. Moreover, it has a higher risk of failure (~10%) due to anatomical variations, necessitating repeat injections. Moreover, IAN blocks may be associated with a higher risk of local and systemic complications such as haematoma formation followed by trismus, damage to IAN, transient facial palsy due to accidental injection close to the parotid gland, as well as intravascular injection which increases the risk of cardiovascular side effects and toxicity. There is growing evidence that infiltration with articaine can be as effective as an IAN block allowing effective pain control during invasive dental procedures in the posterior mandible without the risks of complications. This is discussed in more detail later.

Dental injections provoke stress, fear and anxiety amongst patients, and dentists must manage patients' concerns through frequent reassurance, empathy, effective communication and use of appropriate distraction techniques. Routine use of topical anaesthesia, slow administration of LA (~30 seconds per mL of LA) and allowing adequate time for LA to become effective (3–5 minutes) are fundamental to ensure a positive patient experience. Moreover, medical emergencies which may be precipitated by stress and anxiety (e.g., vasovagal fainting) are more likely to happen prior to or during LA administration. It is recommended to administer all LA injections including IAN blocks with the patient in supine position to ensure adequate cerebral perfusion in the patient. Supine patient position also provides improved access to the injection site for the dentist.

3.2 LOCAL ANAESTHETICS USED IN DENTISTRY

The key requirements for local anaesthetics in dentistry include rapid onset of action, effective pain control, adequate duration of action (30–60 minutes) and shelflife. The actions should be completely reversible without any risk of permanent changes in the nerves, and there. Moreover, the risks of side effects such as systemic toxicity, allergy and addiction should be low. Local anaesthetics used in contemporary clinical dental practice fulfil most of these requirements.

Clinical Dental Pharmacology, First Edition. Edited by Kamran Ali.
© 2024 John Wiley & Sons Ltd. Published 2024 by John Wiley & Sons Ltd.

Table 3.1   Classification of Local Anaesthetics

Esters	Amides
Esters of benzoic acid	Lignocaine (Lidocaine)
Cocaine	Mepivacaine
Butacaine	Prilocaine
Benzocaine	Articaine
Piperocaine	Ropivacaine
Tetracaine	Cinchocaine
Esters of para-amino benzoic acid (PABA)	
Procaine	
Chloroprocaine	
Proxproxycaine	

3.2.1 CLASSIFICATION

Local anaesthetics used in dentistry are classified as esters or amides (Table 3.1). Injectable local anaesthetics used in contemporary dentistry belong exclusively to the amide group due to their superior properties such as, rapid onset of action, improved pain control, longer duration of action, and lower risk of allergy and other side effects compared to the ester-type local anaesthetics. Nevertheless, ester-based local anaesthetics continue to be used for topical (surface) anaesthesia.

Once absorbed into the systemic circulation, the ester-type local anaesthetics are hydrolysed by the enzyme pseudocholinesterase in the blood plasma. The amide-type local anaesthetics are metabolised primarily in the liver. Both types of local anaesthetics are excreted through the kidneys. Impaired renal function can reduce the excretion of local anaesthetics and their metabolites, increasing the risk of toxicity.

3.2.2 VASOCONSTRICTORS

The oral cavity is richly vascularised, and it is common to use local anaesthetics with vasoconstrictors in clinical dentistry. They serve the following purposes:

i. Counter the vasodilatory effects of local anaesthetics and reduce their systemic absorption. This action helps to localise the drug to the site of administration and keep the plasma levels of the drug low, thereby minimising the risk of toxicity.

ii. The local anaesthetics remain localised to the site of injection in higher amounts and for longer, increasing their duration of action.

iii. Reduce bleeding at the operative site which improves access during surgical procedures and facilitates haemostasis.

Vasoconstrictors are added in very low concentrations in dental local anaesthetic solutions. The most common vasoconstrictor used is adrenaline (epinephrine), and its dilution is expressed as a ratio. The most common dilutions of adrenaline are shown as follows:

- 1:80,000 equivalent to 0.0125 mg/mL (12.5 µg/mL)

- 1:100,000 equivalent to 0.01 mg/mL (10 µg/mL)

- 1:200,000 equivalent to 0.05 mg/mL (5 µg/mL)

Local anaesthetics containing vasoconstrictors need to be acidified to prevent oxidation of the vasopressor. Sodium bisulphite is the most common antioxidant used in local anaesthetics for this purpose. Plain local anaesthetics have a pH of 5.5–6.5, but local anaesthetics with adrenaline have a pH of 3.0–5.5. The acidification of local anaesthetics containing adrenaline results in a slower onset of action (due to higher proportion of RNH$^+$ as explained later) and may also produce a burning sensation on injection. Nevertheless, the benefits of adrenaline overweight these disadvantages.

Although local anaesthetics containing adrenaline continue to be used in contemporary dentistry, clinicians should be aware of the potential effects and risks and should take appropriate measures to prevent complications associated with adrenaline. Intravascular administration local anaesthetics containing adrenaline can result in tachycardia (manifested as pounding in the chest or palpitations), an increase in blood pressure and sweating and may even lead to disturbances in heart rhythm in susceptible patients. Moreover, intravascular injection results in systemic distribution of the local anaesthetic drug, rendering the injection ineffective. Clinicians must take appropriate precautions to prevent these complications. These include the following:

- Avoid intravascular injection by using reliable methods of aspiration prior to administration of an injection.

- Administer injections slowly administering using the minimal volume of local anaesthetic (see Section 3.5).

- Observe the patient throughout the injection.

- Maintain communication with the patient and stop the injection should the patient develop palpitations or become unwell.

Local anaesthetics containing adrenaline are generally safe when used appropriately. Patients with a history of mild to moderate cardiovascular disease (ASA II or III) can also receive up to 4 mL of local anaesthetics with adrenaline provided they are in a stable state. In any case, elective dental treatment should not be undertaken in general dental practice settings for patients with uncontrolled hypertension or unstable angina or ASA IV cardiovascular disease.

Local anaesthetics containing adrenaline are contraindicated in patients with hyperthyroidism and those taking non-selective β blockers, such as propranolol, pindolol, sotalol and timolol. Administration of adrenaline in patients taking non-selective β blockers carriers a risk of marked elevation of blood pressure and reflex bradycardia. Patients taking tricyclic antidepressants are also at an increased of developing dysrhythmias with adrenaline, and the dose of local anaesthetic with adrenaline 1:80,000 should be limited to 4 mL in a single appointment.

A large dose of local anaesthetics containing adrenaline should be avoided on the palate as it can lead to ischaemic necrosis of the palatal mucosa (Figure 3.1).

Apart from adrenaline, other vasoconstrictors used in dental anaesthetic solutions include the following:

- *Felypressin* is used in a dilution of 0.03 IU/mL in combination with 3% prilocaine. It has oxytocic properties, and there is a theoretical risk of stimulation of uterine contractions. Therefore, it should be avoided in pregnant women. It is a suitable alternative if there is a contraindication to the use of a local anaesthetic with adrenaline.

- *Levonordefrin* is used in a dilution of 1:20,000 in combination with 2% mepivacaine. Its effects are similar to adrenaline but only 15% as potent.

3.2.3 MECHANISM OF ACTION

Local anaesthetics produce a transient and reversible blockage of impulse conduction in nerve axons and other excitable membranes. The sensation of pain is affected first followed warmth, cold, touch and deep pressure. The effects of local anaesthetics are achieved by a reduction in the

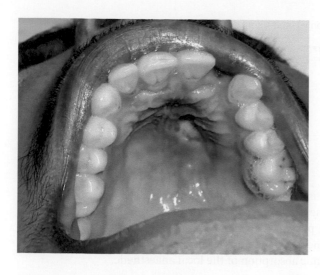

FIGURE 3.1   Ischaemic necrosis of the left palatal mucosa following injection of lignocaine with adrenaline

permeability of sodium channels across nerve membranes. This increases the threshold for nerve excitation and slows the propagation of nerve impulses.

Local anaesthetics are only effective as long as they present at the site of injection. Once absorbed from the site of administration into the systemic circulation, local anaesthetics will no longer provide pain control.

Most local anaesthetics for clinical use in dentistry are available as hydrochloride salts. These salts are water-soluble and stable[1]. When dissolved in sterile water or saline, the local anaesthetic salts exist in two forms simultaneously:

  i. Uncharged molecules or base denoted by RN

  ii. Positively charged molecules or cations denoted by RNH^+

The relative proportion of the base and cations is influenced by the pH of the anaesthetic solution and tissues into which it is injected. When the pH is low (acidic) most of the solution exists as cations, whereas at a higher pH (alkaline) the free base dominates.

Acidic pH	$RNH^+ > RN + H^+$
Alkaline pH	$RNH^+ < RN + H^+$

In addition, the relative proportion of the base and cations is influenced by the dissociation constant (pK_a) of individual local anaesthetics. pK_a measures the affinity of the anaesthetic for hydrogen ions. If the pH of the solution is the same as the pK_a of the local anaesthetic, the relative proportions of RNH^+ and RN+ are equal, i.e., 50% each.

3.2.4 ONSET OF ACTION

The onset of action of local anaesthetics is influenced by several factors as summarised in Table 3.2.

- *pK_a of a local anaesthetic*: If the pK_a of a local anaesthetic is low, RN molecules dominate, allowing rapid diffusion through the nerve sheath which translates to a more rapid onset of action.

- *Lipid solubility*: Increased lipid solubility of a local anaesthetic enhances its diffusion through the nerve membrane, resulting in a more rapid onset and greater potency.

Table 3.2 Properties of Commonly Used Local Anaesthetics in Dentistry

Local anaesthetic	pK_a (36 °C)	Lipid solubility	Onset
Lignocaine	7.7	4.0	Moderate
Mepivacaine	7.9	1.0	Moderate
Prilocaine	7.7	1.5	Moderate
Articaine	7.8	17	Moderate

Source: Adapted from Malamed.[1]

- *pH of the target tissues*: If the target tissues are infected or inflamed, the onset of the local anaesthetic is delayed and its effectiveness is reduced for several reasons. Firstly, during inflammation, the tissue pH drops from the physiologic value of 7.4 to below 6 which reduces the diffusion of local anaesthetics across the nerve membrane. Secondly, the increased vascularity of inflamed tissues increases the systemic absorption of the local anaesthetic.

3.2.5 DURATION OF ACTION

The duration of action is influenced by several factors including the following:

- Accuracy of injection technique, especially for an IAN block.

- *Presence of vasoconstrictor in local anaesthetic*: Addition of vasoconstrictors (e.g., adrenaline) in the local anaesthetic solution increases the duration of action.

- *Vascularity of tissue*: Inflammation at the site of infection results in more rapid absorption of the drug and reduces the duration of action.

- *Protein binding*: Increased binding of the anaesthetic to the protein receptors in the target tissues delays their removal and increases the duration of action.

- *Type of injection*: Nerve blocks usually provide a longer (almost double) duration of both pulpal and soft tissue anaesthesia compared to drugs administered by infiltration.

- Individual variations in response to the drug(s) injected; in most patients, the duration of action is predictable. The duration of action may be too short (hypo-responders) or too long (hyper-responders) in a minority of patients. However, this cannot be predicted reliably the first time a dentist administers LA to a new patient, though one may have a fair idea following repeated episodes of treatment under LA on the same patient.

Table 3.3 summarises the mean duration of action of commonly used local anaesthetics in dentistry, both with and without a vasoconstrictor.

3.3 INJECTABLE LOCAL ANAESTHETICS

3.3.1 LIGNOCAINE (LIDOCAINE) HCl

Lignocaine was the first amide local anaesthetic to replace procaine in 1948, and since then it continues to be the most widely used local anaesthetic. Lignocaine is marketed as hydrochloride salt and is supplied as a 2% solution (20 mg/mL) with and without a vasoconstrictor. Lignocaine causes vasodilation which leads it its rapid absorption in the systemic circulation. Plain lignocaine

Table 3.3   Duration of Commonly Used Local Anaesthetics in Dentistry

Local anaesthetic	Pulpal anaesthesia (minutes)	Soft tissue anaesthesia (minutes)
Lignocaine		
2% plain	5–10	60–120
2% with adrenaline 1:80,000	~60	180–300
Mepivacaine		
3% plain	20–40	120–180
2% with adrenaline 1:200,000	~60	120–300
2% with levonordefrin 1:20,000	60	180–300
Prilocaine		
4% plain	10–15	90–120
4% with adrenaline 1:200,000	60–90	180–480
Articaine		
4% with adrenaline 1:100,000	60–75	180–360
4% with adrenaline 1:200,000	45–60	120–300

Source: Adapted from Malamed.[1]

(pH = 6.5) has a duration of action limited to 5–10 minutes with infiltrations and 10–20 minutes with nerve blocks which renders it unsuitable for routine use in dentistry. Lignocaine 2% with adrenaline 1:80,000/1:100,000 (pH = 5.0–5.5) is preferred over the plain form for most dental procedures. The duration of anaesthesia with lignocaine containing adrenaline is summarised in Table 3.3.

***COMMERCIAL PREPARATIONS*:**

- *Lignospan special*: 2% lidocaine (20 mg/mL) with 1:80,000 (12.5 µg/mL) adrenaline (epinephrine)

- *Lignospan*® *Standard*: 2% lidocaine (20 mg/mL) with 1:100,000 (10 µg/mL) adrenaline (epinephrine)

- *Xylocaine*® *Standard*: 2% lidocaine (20 mg/mL) with 1:80,000 (12.5 µg/mL) adrenaline (epinephrine)

- *Xylocaine*®: 2% lidocaine (20 mg/mL) with 1:100,000 (10 µg/mL) adrenaline (epinephrine)

- *Xylocaine*®: Plain 2% lidocaine (20 mg/mL)

3.3.2 MEPIVACAINE HCl

Mepivacaine is an amide and is marketed as a hydrochloride salt. It is supplied as a 3% solution (30 mg/mL) without a vasoconstrictor (pH = 4.5). It causes mild vasodilation, and the duration of anaesthesia with plain mepivacaine is up to 20 minutes after infiltrations and up to 40 minutes after nerve blocks. Plain mepivacaine is useful for patients in whom use of a vasoconstrictor is contraindicated or unsafe.

Mepivacaine 2% (20 mg/mL) with adrenaline (1:100,000) as well as levonordefrin (1:20,000) is also available (pH = 3.0–3.5). The duration of anaesthesia with mepivacaine containing vasoconstrictors is summarised in Table 3.3.

COMMERCIAL PREPARATIONS:

- Scandonest® plain 3% mepivacaine (30 mg/mL)

- Scandonest® Special 2% mepivacaine (20 mg/mL) with 1:100,000 (10 µg/mL) adrenaline (epinephrine)

- Scandonest® 2% mepivacaine (20 mg/mL) with 1:20,000 (50 µg/mL) levonordefrin

3.3.3 PRILOCAINE HCl

Prilocaine is an amide and is marketed as a hydrochloride salt. It is supplied as a 3% solution (30 mg/mL) or 4% solution (40 mg/mL) without a vasoconstrictor (pH = 4.5). The duration of anaesthesia with plain mepivacaine is 10–15 minutes after infiltrations and 40–60 minutes after nerve blocks. It is also available as 3% solution (30 mg/mL) with felypressin 0.03 IU/mL and 4% solution (40 mg/mL) with adrenaline 1:200,000 (pH = 3.0–4.0). The duration of anaesthesia with prilocaine containing adrenaline is summarised in Table 3.3.

Prilocaine is hydrolysed by hepatic amidases into *ortho*-toluidine and *N*-propylalanine along with the production of carbon dioxide as a byproduct. *Ortho*-toluidine can induce the formation of methaemoglobin with a risk of methaemoglobinemia. Iron in the haemoglobin molecule is continuously converted from the ferrous (reduced) form to the ferric (oxidised) form – referred to as methaemoglobin. The ferric form binds firmly to oxygen in the haemoglobin, preventing its release to the cells. Normally, the level of methaemoglobin is maintained below 1% by the enzyme methaemoglobin reductase. An overdose of prilocaine in susceptible patients can increase the formation of methaemoglobin, which is characterised by cyanosis and may lead to respiratory depression. Prilocaine should be avoided in patients with congenital methaemoglobinemia or other conditions associated with reduced oxygen-carrying capacity of blood. Methaemoglobinemia is treated with intravenous infusion of 1% methylene blue which accepts electrons and facilitates the conversion of iron in ferric form to ferrous form.

COMMERCIAL PREPARATIONS:

- Citanest® plain 4% prilocaine (40 mg/mL)

- Citanest® Forte 4% prilocaine (40 mg/mL) with 1:200,000 (5 µg/mL) adrenaline (epinephrine)

- Citanest® with octapressin 3% prilocaine (30 mg/mL) with 0.03 IU/mL (30 µg/mL) felypressin

3.3.4 ARTICAINE HCl

Articaine is an amide and is marketed as a hydrochloride salt. It is the only amide-type local anaesthetic which also contains an ester group. Therefore, biotransformation of articaine occurs via two pathways, i.e., hydrolysis by plasma esterase and degradation by hepatic microsomal enzymes.

Articaine causes vasodilation similar to lignocaine. It is supplied as a 4% solution (40 mg/mL) with adrenaline 1:100,000 (pH = 4.4–5.2) or 1:200,000 (pH = 4.6–5.4). The duration of anaesthesia with articaine containing adrenaline is summarised in Table 3.3.

Articaine has a higher lipid solubility and offers an advantage of higher bone penetration compared to other commonly used local anaesthetics in dentistry. There is growing evidence that buccal infiltration with articaine can provide adequate anaesthesia of palatal soft tissues avoiding the need for painful palatal injections in procedures such as tooth extractions[2, 3]. Similarly, infiltration injections with articaine in the mandibular molar/premolar region can obviate the need for an

IAN block during procedures such as endodontics and tooth extractions and avoid the challenges and complications associated with IAN blocks.[4–6]

COMMERCIAL PREPARATIONS:

- *Septanest*: 4% articaine (40 mg/mL) with 1:100,000 (10 μg/mL) adrenaline (epinephrine)
- *Septanest*: 4% articaine (40 mg/mL) with 1:200,000 (5 μg/mL) adrenaline (epinephrine)
- *Septocaine*®: 4% articaine (40 mg/mL) with 1:100,000 (10 μg/mL) adrenaline (epinephrine)
- *Septocaine*®: 4% articaine (40 mg/mL) with 1:200,000 (5 μg/mL) adrenaline (epinephrine)

3.4 LOCAL ANAESTHETICS FOR TOPICAL (SURFACE) USE

Topical anaesthetics are important for painless administration of local anaesthetic injections and also serve to reassure the patient prior to penetration with a needle. Topical agents anaesthetise the surface tissue to a depth of 2–3 mm and serve to minimise the discomfort associated with a needle prick.

All local anaesthetics (except cocaine) cause variable degree of vasodilation. Topical agents do not contain a vasoconstrictor and are typically used in higher concentrations to facilitate diffusion across the mucosa/skin. These factors can lead to rapid absorption in the systemic circulation increasing the risk of toxicity comparable to local anaesthetics administered intravenously. Some of the most commonly used topical local anaesthetics used in dentistry include the following:

3.4.1 ESTER-BASED TOPICAL AGENTS

Ester-based agents are effective topical agents, but dental clinicians should recognise that they carry a recognised risk of allergy and warrant appropriate precautions.

- Ultracare® Benzocaine gel (75, 100, 150, 180 and 200 mg/mL)
- *Cetacaine*® *Benzocaine, Butamben and Tetracaine HCl*: contains benzocaine 14% (140 mg/mL), butamben 2% (20 mg/mL) and tetracaine hydrochloride 2% (20 mg/mL); available as aerosol, gel, ointment and solution

3.4.2 AMIDE-BASED TOPICAL AGENTS

Aerosol 1% (10 mg/metred spray)

Ointment 5% (50 mg/mL)

Solution 2.5% (25 mg/mL); 4% (40 mg/mL)

Patch (46.1 mg/patch)

Xylonor gel 2% (20 mg/g); 5% (50 mg/g)

Xylonor® spray 10% (100 mg/mL) 15% (150 mg/mL)

- *EMLA (eutectic mixture of local anaesthetics)*: contains 2.5% lignocaine and 2.5% prilocaine in an emulsion in a 1:1 by weight. It is supplied in a tube or as an EMLA anaesthetic disc. EMLA is used for surface anaesthesia of the skin prior to needle injection/venepuncture. It is contraindicated in patients with congenital methaemoglobinemia as well as infants (<1 year)

3.5 DOSAGE LIMITS

The dose limits of local anaesthetic drugs are summarised in Table 3.4. Given that most types of dental treatment can be undertaken with minimal volume of LA, i.e., 0.6 mL for infiltration and 1.5 mL for an IAN block, these limits should not be reached. If adequate anaesthesia is not achieved after repeating the injection 2–3 times, the clinician must re-evaluate the factors which may be responsible for failure of anaesthesia before attempting further injection(s).

The manufacturers recommend higher absolute maximum dose limits for local anaesthetics with a vasoconstrictor as the presence of a vasoconstrictor reduces systemic absorption of the drug. However, the dose limits presented here are not adjusted for the presence of a vasoconstrictor in the interest of patient safety, as recommended by the Council of Dental Therapeutics of the American Dental Association.[1] As shown in Table 3.5, these dosage limits translate into 6–7 cartridges for most local anaesthetics and should be more than adequate for most types of dental treatment. It should be noted that the volume of local anaesthetic cartridges for dental use varies with the manufacturers and usually ranges from 1.8 to 2.2 mL. Dental practitioners must consider the volume of local anaesthetic cartridge when calculating the dose as shown in Table 3.5.

It is particularly important to be aware about the increased risk of overdosage in children and elderly. Moreover, LA dose should be reduced in medically compromised patients such as those with compromised hepatic and renal function.

3.5.1 OVERDOSE

Overdose of local anaesthetics is usually results from excessive doses, and the potential for toxicity mainly rests with the user (dental clinician administering the LA). Overdose can be prevented by considering the following:

- Routine dental procedures usually require a low dose of local anaesthetics, and the upper limit of recommended dose should not be approached.

- Particular care is required in children and elderly and those with a history of hepatorenal disease.

Table 3.4   Maximum Dosage of Commonly Used Local Anaesthetics in Dentistry

Maximum recommended dose	Absolute maximum recommended dose
Lignocaine: 4.4 mg/kg	300 mg
Mepivacaine: 6.6 mg/kg	300 mg
Prilocaine: 6.0 mg/kg	400 mg
Articaine: 7 mg/kg	500 mg

Table 3.5   Local Anaesthetic Dose in Milligrams Per Dental Cartridge

Local anaesthetic	mg/mL	1.8 mL cartridge mg/cartridge	2 mL cartridge mg/cartridge	2.2 mL cartridge mg/cartridge
2% Lignocaine	20	36	40	44
2% Mepivacaine	20	36	40	44
3% Mepivacaine	30	54	60	66
3% Prilocaine	30	54	60	66
4% Prilocaine	40	72	80	88
4% Articaine	40	72	80	88

- Caution is also required in patients taking certain medications which may potentiate the effects of local anaesthetics, including meperidine, quinidine, desipramine and cimetidine.

- Treatment of patients requiring multiple procedures should be undertaken in stages rather than in a single appointment.

- Appropriate precautions should be taken to prevent intravascular injections during administration of LA to prevent a rapid rise in plasma levels of local anaesthetics.

- Administration of local anaesthetics should be avoided without a vasoconstrictor.

Mild overdose of local anaesthetics leads to an excitatory response manifested by light headedness, nervousness, visual and auditory disturbances, circumoral numbness, talkativeness, excitation, euphoria, apprehension, slurring of speech, dysarthria, and a rise in heart rate, blood pressure and respiratory rate. Mild overdose is managed with reassurance, oxygen administration and monitoring of vital signs.

Severe overdose may lead to the development of tonic-clonic seizures followed by central nervous system (CNS) depression with a drop in the heart rate, respiratory rate and blood pressure with potential loss of consciousness. Severe overdose requires emergency medical support, and if the patient develops convulsions, they need to be protected. Loss of consciousness with cardiorespiratory arrest requires basic life support until medical help arrives.

3.5.2 ALLERGY

True allergy to amide-type local anaesthetics is exceedingly rare. Contemporary local anaesthetic cartridges are free of latex. Moreover, ingredient, such as methylparaben which was used as a preservative in local anaesthetics and was associated with allergic reactions, is no longer included in local anaesthetic solutions.

Allergic reactions are more likely with ester-type local anaesthetics which are still used for topical anaesthesia. Allergic reactions can manifest as dermatitis, bronchospasm triggered by an asthmatic attack and life-threatening anaphylaxis. Appropriate precautions are required to prevent allergic reactions in susceptible patients, including a thorough medical history and patch testing if required. Recognition and management of anaphylaxis is discussed in the chapter on medical emergencies (Chapter 17).

3.6 SUMMARY

Local anaesthetic injections are a stressful experience for most patients and provoke fear and anxiety and can be associated with a wide range of complications and medicolegal issues. Dental clinicians must consider the following points for safe and effective administration of LA. Meticulous attention to detail is crucial to minimise the risk of local and systemic complications and avoid medicolegal complaints.

- *Pre-anaesthetic assessment*
  - Carefully review patient's medical history to identify any issues which may increase the risk of medical emergencies, cardiorespiratory complications, allergy or overdose.
  - Ensure that all clinical staff are up to date with their training in the management of medical emergencies and cardio-pulmonary resuscitation.
  - Determine the cooperation level of the patient and obtain a valid, informed consent from the patient prior to attempting administration of LA.
  - Reassure the patient, explain the procedure of local anaesthetic administration and work out hand signs to stop the procedure should the patient become unwell.

- *Anaesthetic administration*
  - Recline the dental chair to place the patient in a supine position during anaesthetic administration. This ensures adequate venous return and minimises the risk of a vasovagal syncope.
  - Ensure the patient has appropriate eye protection to prevent accidental eye injuries.
  - Apply a topical anaesthetic to minimise the discomfort associated with needle penetration and wait for at least 1 minute before administering an injection.
  - Assemble the local anaesthetic injection and ensure it is working appropriately before attempting an injection.
  - Keep the injection syringe out of patient's line of sight at all times.
  - Advise the patient to focus on their breathing and flexing their toes during administration of the anaesthetic injection (useful distraction technique to minimise perceived discomfort with local anaesthetic injections and help maintain circulation).
  - Always observe the patient during administering LA and identify any signs indicative of a medical emergency.
  - Avoid intravascular injection by using reliable methods of aspiration prior to administration of an injection.
  - Use appropriate anatomical landmarks and techniques to administer specific injections.
  - Administer injections slowly and inject the minimal volume of local anaesthetic (0.4–0.6 mL over 15–30 seconds for infiltrations and 1.5 mL for IAN block over 30–60 seconds).
  - Never leave the patient unattended after an injection as adverse reactions may develop several minutes after the local anaesthetic administration.
  - Ensure that the local anaesthetic is fully effective before commencing operative treatment. Wait for 2–3 minutes after infiltration(s) and 3–5 minutes after a nerve block to allow the local anaesthetic to become fully effective. Effectiveness of LA should be assessed both subjectively and objectively.
  - Nerve blocks, especially an IAN block, may take some time before they are fully effective. Therefore, wait for at least 5 minutes before administering a repeat IAN block.
  - When administering an IAN block, there is usually no need to administer additional drug for anaesthesia of the lingual nerve. Both the inferior alveolar and lingual nerves are located in the pterygomandibular space, and administration of an IAN block is usually adequate to anaesthetise the lingual nerve.

- *After treatment completion*
  - After the treatment is complete, provide appropriate instructions regarding precautions related to the effects of LA, i.e., patient may experience numbness for up to 2–3 hours, and they should avoid hot food or drinks and also avoid biting their lips, tongue and cheeks during this period.
  - Record contemporaneous clinical notes to include details related to the composition of the local anaesthetic (e.g., 2% lignocaine with adrenaline 1:80,000), type of injection(s) administered (e.g., buccal infiltration/nerve block), volume of the anaesthetic drug administered and the batch number/expiry date of the local anaesthetic cartridge(s) used.
  - Document any complications encountered during the appointment and measures taken to manage those complications.

ACKNOWLEDGEMENTS

Figure 3.1 is provided by Dr Omer Janjua, Allied Hospital Faisalabad, Pakistan.

RESOURCES

RESOURCES FOR DENTAL PROFESSIONALS

American Dental Association. Anesthesia and Sedation. https://www.ada.org/en/resources/research/science-and-research-institute/oral-health-topics/anesthesia-and-sedation (accessed 25 February 2024).

American Academy of Paediatric Dentistry (AAPD). Use of local anesthesia for pediatric dental patient. https://www.aapd.org/globalassets/media/policies_guidelines/bp_localanesthesia.pdf (accessed 25 February 2024).

RESOURCES FOR DENTAL PATIENTS

Healthline. What you need to know about dental anesthesia. https://www.healthline.com/health/dental-and-oral-health/dental-anesthesia (accessed 25 February 2024).

REFERENCES

1. Malamed, S.F. (2013). *Handbook of Local Anesthesia*, 6e. Elsevier: 314 p.

2. Gholami, M., Banihashemrad, A., Mohammadzadeh, A., and Ahrari, F. (2021). The efficacy of 4% articaine versus 2% lidocaine in inducing palatal anesthesia for tooth extraction in different maxillary regions. *Journal of Oral and Maxillofacial Surgery* 79 (8): 1643–1649.

3. Abdul Kalam Azad (2018). NCT03470532. Comparing articaine and mepivacaine without palatal injection in pain assessment during maxillary teeth extraction. https://clinicaltrials.gov/show/nct03470532 (accessed 27 September 2023).

4. Venkat Narayanan, J., Gurram, P., Krishnan, R. et al. (2017). Infiltrative local anesthesia with articaine is equally as effective as inferior alveolar nerve block with lidocaine for the removal of erupted molars. *Oral and Maxillofacial Surgery* 21 (3): 295–299.

5. Yang, F., Gao, Y., Zhang, L. et al. (2020). Local anaesthesia for surgical extraction of mandibular third molars: a systematic review and network meta-analysis. *Clinical Oral Investigations* 24 (11): 3781–3800.

6. Yu, J., Liu, S., and Zhang, X. (2021). Can buccal infiltration of articaine replace traditional inferior alveolar nerve block for the treatment of mandibular molars in pediatric patients?: a systematic review and meta-analysis. *Medicina Oral, Patología Oral y Cirugía Bucal* 26 (6): e754.

Antimicrobial Medications

Use of Antibiotics in Dentoalveolar Infections

Kamran Ali

Qatar University, QU Health, College of Dental Medicine, Doha, Qatar

4.1 INTRODUCTION

Dentoalveolar infections most commonly result from spread of infection from dental pulp into the periradicular tissues and may manifest in the form of a dentoalveolar abscess. Untreated/aggressive periradicular infection may lead to a spreading cellulitis or even osteomyelitis of jaw bones. Apart from pulp infection secondary to untreated caries or trauma, dentoalveolar infection may result also from surgical interventions, especially in immunocompromised patients. Infections of periodontal origin are discussed separately in Chapter 4.

Most dentoalveolar infections are localised and can be managed with appropriate operative measures such as root canal treatment or extraction of the involved tooth and do not warrant antibiotic prescriptions[1, 2]. However, periradicular infection may spread further through the fascial planes and lead to involvement of the upper airways, and periorbital tissues with risk of further spread to the eyeball and brain[3]. Spreading cellulitis secondary to dental and oral infection is extremely painful and associated marked systemic involvement with fever, malaise, lymphadenopathy, difficulty in swallowing, airway compression and dehydration. Spreading cellulitis of odontogenic origin may be complicated by airway compression and sepsis with a potentially fatal outcome[4].

Historically, antibiotics have been used widely in the management of dentoalveolar infections. However, antibiotic resistance, discussed in Chapter 6, is a major global health threat with growing magnitude and warrants evidence-based and judicious use of antibiotics[4]. In addition, antibiotics, like other drugs, are associated with adverse reactions and entail a financial cost. Therefore, antibiotics should only be prescribed when necessary and consideration should be given to the patients' medical history, concurrent medications, and risk of drug interactions. The aim of this chapter is to discuss appropriate use of antibiotics in contemporary clinical dentistry.

4.1.1 PRINCIPLES OF ANTIBIOTIC PRESCRIPTION IN DENTISTRY

- Most dental problems are best managed with local measures involving operative dental treatment; antibiotics do not compensate for inadequate operative dental treatment.

- Prescribe antibiotics only when indicated.

- The decision to prescribe antibiotics should be informed by clinical findings and should not be based on patient's request.

- Most odontogenic infections are caused by a mixed bacterial population, appropriate antibiotics may be prescribed blindly, and non-resolving infections may require culture and sensitivity of causative microorganism in hospital settings.

Clinical Dental Pharmacology, First Edition. Edited by Kamran Ali.
© 2024 John Wiley & Sons Ltd. Published 2024 by John Wiley & Sons Ltd.

- First-line antibiotics used in the management of dentoalveolar infections include phenoxymethylpenicillin, amoxicillin and metronidazole. Alternate options include co-amoxiclav, clindamycin, azithromycin and clarithromycin.

- Most antibiotics in dental settings are administered orally.

- The duration of therapy ranges from 3 to 7 days, most commonly antibiotics are prescribed for 5 days.

- When prescribing an antibiotic, consider the patient's medical history including any allergies and concurrent medications to evaluate risk of adverse effects, cautions and drug interactions.

Antibiotics not Indicated

- Pulpitis

- Apical periodontitis

- Localised dentoalveolar abscess

- Alveolar osteitis (dry socket)

- Mild pericoronitis

- Uncomplicated endodontics and tooth extractions in medically fit and healthy patients.

Antibiotics Indicated

Antibiotics may be used an adjunct to operative interventions to manage the following conditions:

- Rapidly progressive diffuse swelling involving fascial spaces

- Poorly localised dentoalveolar abscess

- Dental infection associated with severe trismus (<10 mm inter-incisal opening)

- Severe pericoronitis (with systemic features)

- Osteomyelitis

- Maxillary sinusitis complicating an oroantral communication/fistula

It needs to be reiterated that patients presenting with features of a spreading cellulitis and systemic involvement often require a comprehensive management including intravenous antibiotics, parenteral analgesia, supportive therapy and close monitoring of vital signs. Management of such patients with oral antibiotics in outpatient dental settings may not be appropriate and such patients need to be referred to oral and maxillofacial surgery at a local hospital for management as in-patients[5]. The indications for urgent referral to oral and maxillofacial surgery are summarised in Table 4.1.

Table 4.1 Indications for Urgent Referral of Patients with Dentoalveolar Infections

- Difficulty in breathing/swallowing
- Severe trismus (<10 mm)
- Swelling extending beyond the alveolar process
- Elevated temperature (>102 °F)
- Severe malaise or toxic appearance
- Compromised host defences
- Need for treatment under general anaesthesia

Table 4.2   Red and Amber Flags of Sepsis

Red flags	Amber flags
• New deterioration in GCS/AVPU • Systolic BP ≤90 mmHg (or ≥40 mmHg below normal) • Heart rate > 130 per minute • Respiratory rate ≥ 25 per minute • Requires oxygen to keep SpO$_2$ 92% (88% in COPD) • Non-blanching rash or mottled/ashen/cyanotic • Not passed urine in the last 18 hours • Recent chemotherapy (within the last 6 weeks)	• Relatives worried about mental state/behaviour • Acute deterioration in functional ability • Immunosuppressed (without recent chemotherapy) • Trauma, surgery or procedure in the last 6 weeks • Respiratory rate 21–24 or dyspnoeic • Systolic BP 91–100 mmHg • Heart rate 91–130 or new dysrhythmia • Not passed urine in the last 12–18 hours • Tympanic temperature ≤ 36 °C • Clinical signs of wound, device or skin infection

Moreover, dentoalveolar infections may be complicated by sepsis which could be potentially life-threatening. Sepsis is characterised by organ dysfunction and may result from an imbalanced reaction of the body to an infection and is associated with a recognised risk of multiple organ failure and mortality. The UK sepsis trust has provided guidelines on recognition of red and amber flags of sepsis in patients with suspected signs and symptoms of infections (Table 4.2)[6]. Although sepsis of dental origin is rare, patients with dentoalveolar infections with features of sepsis should be referred urgently to a local hospital for prompt assessment and management[7].

4.2 COMMON ANTIBIOTICS USED IN DENTOALVEOLAR INFECTIONS

A wide range of antibiotics are used in medical practice and include both bactericidal and bacteriostatic agents. However, management of dentoalveolar infections involves use of a narrow range of antibiotics. The most commonly used antibiotics are discussed in below.

4.2.1 PENICILLINS (PENAMS)

Penicillins are a group of bactericidal antibiotics and are one of the most widely used antibiotics in dentistry. Penicillins (and cephalosporins) are referred to as β-lactam antibiotics because of their unique four-membered lactam ring. Hypersensitivity reactions are a well-recognised side effect of penicillins.

Mechanism of action: Penicillins inhibit bacterial cell wall synthesis by combining with the transpeptidase responsible for cross-linking of the peptidoglycan; activity depends on an intact β-lactam ring. Common types of penicillins used in dentistry are mentioned in the following section:

Phenoxymethylpenicillin (Penicillin V)

This is an oral penicillin that resists destruction by the gastric acid and often used as a first-line penicillin for dentoalveolar infections due to its narrow spectrum and lower risk of driving antimicrobial resistance.

Cautions: History of allergy, renal impairment.

Contra-indications: Penicillin hypersensitivity.

Side effects: Sensitivity reactions including urticaria, fever, joint pains, angioedema, transient leukopenia and thrombocytopenia, anaphylactic shock, diarrhoea.

COMMERCIAL PREPARATIONS:

Phenoxymethylpenicillin®

Tablets, phenoxy methyl penicillin (as potassium salt) 250 mg.

Oral solution, phenoxymethylpenicillin (as potassium salt) for reconstitution with water, 125 mg/5 mL, 250 mg/5 mL.

ROUTE OF ADMINISTRATION AND DOSE:

By mouth, 500 mg (2 × 250 mg tablets) every 6 hours.

Child every 6 hours up to 1 year 62.5 mg, 1–5 years 125 mg, 6–11 years 250 mg; 12–17 years 500 mg.

Amoxicillin

Amoxicillin is a broad-spectrum penicillin and is absorbed well from the gastrointestinal tract (GIT) producing adequate plasma and tissue concentrations.

Cautions: History of allergy, renal impairment, erythematous rashes common in glandular fever, chronic lymphatic leukaemia and possibly HIV infection.

Contra-indications: Penicillin hypersensitivity.

Side effects: Nausea, diarrhoea, rashes, rarely antibiotic-associated colitis.

COMMERCIAL PREPARATIONS:

Amoxil®

Capsules, amoxicillin (as trihydrate) 250 mg, 500 mg.
Dispersible tablets, amoxicillin (as trihydrate) 125 mg, 250 mg, 500 mg.
Syrup, amoxicillin (as trihydrate), for reconstitution with water 125 mg/5 mL, 250 mg/5 mL.
Paediatric suspension, amoxicillin 125 mg (as trihydrate)/1.25 mL when reconstituted with water.

ROUTE OF ADMINISTRATION AND DOSE:

By mouth, 500 mg every 8 hours. Child every 8 hours 6–11 months 125 mg; 1–4 years 250 mg; 5–11 years 500 mg; 12–17 years 500 mg.

Co Amoxiclav

Co-amoxiclav is a combination of clavulanic acid, an inhibitor of penicillinase, and amoxicillin and may be used as a second-line therapy.

Cautions: Hepatic impairment (monitor hepatic function), pregnancy.

Contra-indications: Penicillin hypersensitivity, history of co-amoxiclav-associated (or penicillin-associated) jaundice or hepatic dysfunction.

Side effects: Hepatitis, cholestatic jaundice, erythema multiforme (including Stevens–Johnson syndrome), toxic epidermal necrolysis, exfoliative dermatitis, vasculitis; rarely prolongation of bleeding, dizziness, headache, convulsions (particularly with high doses and in renal impairment); superficial staining of teeth with suspension.

COMMERCIAL PREPARATIONS:

Augmentin®

Tablets, 375 mg con-amoxiclav 250/125 (amoxicillin 250 mg as trihydrate, clavulanic acid 125 mg as potassium salt).

Tablets, 625 mg con-amoxiclav 500/125 (amoxicillin 500 mg as trihydrate, clavulanic acid 125 mg as potassium salt).

Oral suspension, 120/31, sugar free, co-amoxiclav (amoxicillin 125 mg as trihydrate, clavulanic acid 31 mg as potassium salt)/5 mL when reconstituted with water.

Oral suspension, 250/62, sugar free, co-amoxiclav (amoxicillin 250 mg as trihydrate, clavulanic acid 62 mg as potassium salt)/5 mL when reconstituted with water.

ROUTE OF ADMINISTRATION AND DOSE:

By mouth, expressed as amoxicillin, 250 mg every 8 hours, dose doubled in severe infections.

Child, below 6 years 125/31 suspension 8-hourly; 6–12 years 250/31 suspension 8-hourly.

4.2.2 CEPHALOSPORINS

Cephalosporins are broad-spectrum bactericidal antimicrobials with activity against a wide range of gram-positive and gram-negative bacteria. Like penicillins, cephalosporins also contain a β-lactam ring which is a key component for their antibacterial activity. Antibacterial activity can be altered by variation in the side chains of the cephalosporin nucleus.

Cephalosporins are classified into different generations based on their structure, antimicrobial spectrum, and activity against bacteria, and five generations of cephalosporins are well recognised, each generation had a varying spectrum of activity. The first-generation cephalosporins are primarily effective against gram-positive bacteria, while subsequent generations have an increasing effectiveness against gram-negative bacteria (with reduced activity against gram-positive bacteria) except fourth generation which have extended spectrum against gram-negative and some gram-positive bacteria. Different generations of cephalosporins are summarised in Table 4.3.

Mechanism of action: Cephalosporins are bactericidal and inhibit cell wall synthesis by combining with the transpeptidase responsible for cross-linking of the peptidoglycan; they are stable to many bacterial β-lactamases.

Table 4.3 Classification of Cephalosporins

Cephalosporin generation	Examples
First	Cephazolin, Cephalexin, Cephalothin Cephradine
Second	Cefuroxime, Cefoxitin, Cefaclor, Cefadroxil
Third	Cefotaxime, Ceftazidime, Cefodizime, Ceftriaxone Cefixime, Cefoperazone
Fourth	Cefepime
Fifth	Ceftaroline, Ceftobiprole

Side effects: Apart from gastrointestinal symptoms like nausea, vomiting and diarrhoea, the principal side effect of the cephalosporins is hypersensitivity. Up to 10% patients with sensitivity to penicillins may also be allergic to the cephalosporins. Increased bleeding tendency due to interference with blood clotting factors has been associated with several cephalosporins.

Cephalosporins are not used as the first-line antibiotics in dentoalveolar infections. However, some cephalosporins are recommended for prophylaxis against bacterial endocarditis prior to dental procedures in susceptible patients as an alternative option in some countries including the United States of America (Chapter 6).

Cephalexin

It belongs to first generation of cephalosporins.

Indications: Infections due to sensitive gram-positive and gram-negative bacteria.

Cautions: Penicillin sensitivity; renal impairment; pregnancy and breastfeeding (but appropriate to use); false-positive urinary glucose (if tested for reducing substances) and false-positive (Coombs test).

Contra-indications: Cephalosporin hypersensitivity; porphyria.

Side effects: Diarrhoea, antibiotic-associated colitis (rare) (both more likely with higher doses), nausea, vomiting, abdominal discomfort, headache; rashes, pruritus, urticaria, serum sickness-like reactions, fever, arthralgia anaphylaxis; erythema multiforme, toxic epidermal necrolysis; disturbances in liver enzymes, transient hepatitis and cholestatic jaundice; eosinophilia and blood disorders.

COMMERCIAL PREPARATIONS:

Ceporex®
Capsules, cephalexin 250 mg, 500 mg.
Tablets, f/c cephalexin 250 mg, 500 mg.
Syrup, cephalexin for reconstitution with water, 125 mg/5 mL, 250 mg/5 mL, 500 mg/5 mL.

Keflex®
Capsules, cephalexin 250 mg, 500 mg.
Tablets, f/c cephalexin 250 mg, 500 mg.
Suspension, cephalexin for reconstitution with water, 125 mg/5 mL, 250 mg/5 mL.

ROUTE OF ADMINISTRATION AND DOSE:

By mouth, 250 mg every 6 hours or 500 mg every 8–12 hours increased to 1–1.5 g every 6–8 hours for severe infections. Child, 25 mg/kg daily in divided doses, doubled for severe infections maximum 100 mg/kg; or under 1 year, 125 mg every 12 hours; 1–5 years, 125 mg every 8 hours; 6–12 years 250 mg every 8 hours.

4.2.3 METRONIDAZOLE

Metronidazole belongs to the nitroimidazole class of drugs and has both antibacterial as well as antiprotozoal activity. It is effective against anaerobic bacteria, including bacteroides, anaerobic cocci and clostridia. Bacterial resistance is uncommon.

Mechanism of action: Bactericidal, converted by anaerobic bacteria to active (reduced) metabolite, inhibits DNA synthesis by anaerobic bacteria and protozoa.

Side effects: Nausea, vomiting and metallic taste. Also furred tongue, GIT disturbances; rashes urticaria and angioedema. On prolonged or intensive therapy, peripheral neuropathy, transient epileptic seizures and leukopenia.

Cautions: avoid in patients taking alcohol (Disulfiram-like reaction with alcohol which can present with nausea, vomiting, skin flushing, tachycardia and shortness of breath); avoid in patients taking warfarin; pregnancy and breastfeeding (avoid high-dose regimens).

COMMERCIAL PREPARATIONS:

Metronidazole

Tablets, metronidazole 200 mg, 400 mg.
Suspension, metronidazole (as benzoate) 200 mg/5 mL.

ROUTE OF ADMINISTRATION AND DOSE:

By mouth, 400 mg every 8 hours.

Child, 1–2 years 50 mg 8-hourly; 3–6 years 100 mg 12-hourly; 7–9 years 100 mg 8-hourly; 10–17 years 200 mg 8-hourly.

Topical application

Elyzol® Metronidazole 25% dental gel for application into periodontal pockets as an adjunct to treatment of periodontitis (see Chapter 5).

4.2.4 CLINDAMYCIN

Clindamycin is a lincosamide antibiotic which is primarily bacteriostatic but may have bactericidal effects at high doses. It demonstrates activity against gram-positive cocci, including penicillin-resistant staphylococci and also against many anaerobes, especially *Bacteroides fragilis*. It is well concentrated in bone and excreted in bile and urine.

Mechanism of action: Inhibits protein synthesis by binding to the 50S subunit of the bacterial ribosomes.

Side effects: Diarrhoea (discontinue treatment), abdominal discomfort, nausea, vomiting, antibiotic-associated colitis; jaundice and altered liver function tests; neutropenia, eosinophilia, agranulocytosis and thrombocytopenia reported; rash, urticaria, erythema multiforme, exfoliative and vesiculobullous dermatitis also reported.

Cautions: Clindamycin has only a limited use because of serious side effects. Its most serious toxic effect is antibiotic-associated colitis which may be fatal.

Contra-indications: Diarrhoeal states.

Counselling: If diarrhoea develops, patients should discontinue clindamycin immediately and contact doctor if diarrhoea develops (risk of pseudomembranous colitis); capsules should be swallowed with a glass of water.

COMMERCIAL PREPARATIONS:

Dalacin C
  Capsules, clindamycin (as hydrochloride) 75 mg, 150 mg.
  Oral suspension, clindamycin 75 mg/5 mL.

ROUTE OF ADMINISTRATION AND DOSE:

By mouth, 150 mg every 6 hours; 300 g 6 hourly in severe infections 12–17 years, 150 mg every 6 hours.

4.2.5 MACROLIDES

Macrolides are a group of antibiotics that include erythromycin azithromycin, clarithromycin, spiramycin, dirithromycin and telithromycin.

Mechanism of action: Macrolides inhibit bacterial protein synthesis by binding to the 50S subunit of bacterial ribosomes.

Erythromycin

Erythromycin was the first macrolide antibiotic to be discovered, and historically it has been used as a first-line choice for patients allergic to penicillin. However, erythromycin is used much less frequently in the management of dental infections. This is due to its narrow spectrum (mainly effective against gram-positive bacteria), bacteriostatic activity, significant interactions with other drugs, and emergence of bacterial resistance and the availability of more effective alternatives.

Spectrum: It has a narrow spectrum of activity, similar to that of benzyl penicillin, but is more active against *Staphylococcus aureus* (but not methicillin-resistant strains, MRSA). Also active against *Streptococcus* species (including *Streptococcus pyogenes*, *Streptococcus pneumoniae*). It has limited activity against gram-negative bacteria.

Indications: Historically erythromycin has been used as an alternative to penicillin to treat a variety of respiratory tract infections and also in the prophylaxis against bacterial endocarditis. However, there are limited indications for using erythromycin to treat dentoalveolar infections in the contemporary era.

Side effects: Nausea, vomiting, abdominal discomfort, diarrhoea; urticaria, rashes and other, allergic reactions; reversible hearing loss; cardiac effects (including chest pain and *arrhythmias*).

Contra-indications: Erythromycin estolate is hepatotoxic and is contra-indicated in liver disease.

Cautions: Hepatic and renal impairment; prolongation of QT interval (ventricular tachycardia reported).

COMMERCIAL PREPARATIONS:

Erythrocin®
  Tablets, e/c erythromycin 250 mg, 500 mg.

Erymax®
  Tablets erythromycin stearate 250 mg, 500 mg.

Erythroped®
  Oral suspension, erythromycin (as ethyl succinate) 125 mg/5 mL, 250 mg/5 mL, 500 mg/5 mL.
  Granules, erythromycin (as ethyl succinate), 125 mg/sachet, 250 mg/sachet.

ROUTE OF ADMINISTRATION AND DOSE:

By mouth, adult and child over 8 years, 250–500 mg every 6 hours or 500 mg–1 g every 12 hours; up to 4 g daily in severe infections. Child up to 2 years 125 mg every 6 hours, 2–8 years 250 mg every 6 hours, doses doubled for severe infections.

Azithromycin

Azithromycin is a macrolide antibiotic that have against β-lactamase producing microorganisms. It inhibits many gram-positive aerobic and anaerobic species, a variety of intracellular pathogens, and several aerobic and gram-negative bacteria. It is also used for oral prophylaxis against bacterial endocarditis as an alternative to penicillin.

Side effects: GIT symptoms (nausea, vomiting, diarrhea and abdominal discomfort), hypersensitivity, headache, insomnia, abnormal liver function tests, cholestasis, jaundice, hepatitis and Stevens–Johnson syndrome.

Cautions: Hepatorenal disease, myasthenia gravis; photosensitivity.

COMMERCIAL PREPARATIONS:

Zithromax®

Tablets, azithromycin (as dihydrate) 250 mg, 500 mg.
Oral suspension, azithromycin (as dihydrate) 200 mg/5 mL and 100 mg/5 mL when reconstituted with water.

ROUTE OF ADMINISTRATION AND DOSE:

By mouth, 500 mg once daily for 3 days. Child over 6 months 10 mg/kg once daily for 3 days; or body weight 26–35 kg. 300 mg once daily for 3 days; body weight 36–45 kg, 400 mg once daily for 3 days.

Clarithromycin

Indications: Respiratory tract infections, mild to moderate skin and soft tissue infections; oral prophylaxis against bacterial endocarditis as an alternative to penicillin, adjunct in the treatment of duodenal ulcers by eradication of *Helicobacter pylori*.

Cautions; side effects: See Erythromycin; reduce doses in renal impairment; caution is pregnancy and breast-feeding also reported, headache, taste disturbances, stomatitis, glossitis, cholestasis, jaundice, hepatitis, and Steven's–Johnson syndrome, on intravenous infusion, local tenderness, phlebitis; interactions. In arrhythmias avoid concomitant administration with astemizole or terfenadine; also avoid with cisapride.

COMMERCIAL PREPARATIONS:

Klaricid®
Tablets, f/c clarithromycin 250 mg, 500 mg.
Paediatric suspension, clarithromycin 125 mg/5 mL when reconstituted with water.
Intravenous infusion, powder for reconstitution clarithromycin 500 mg vial.

ROUTE OF ADMINISTRATION AND DOSE:

By mouth, 250 mg every 12 hours for 7 days, increased in severe infections to 500 mg every 12 hours for up to 14 days. Child body weight under 8 kg. 7.5 mg/kg twice daily; 8–11 kg (1–2 years 62.5 mg twice daily; 12–19 kg (3–6 years) 125 mg twice daily; 20–29 kg (7–9 years) 187.56 mg twice daily; 30–40 kg (10–12 years 250 mg twice daily).

RESOURCES

RESOURCES FOR DENTAL PROFESSIONALS

ADA (American Dental Association). Antibiotics for Dental Pain and Swelling Guideline. https://www.ada.org/en/resources/research/science-and-research-institute/evidence-based-dental-research/antibiotics-for-dental-pain-and-swelling (accessed 25 February 2024).

Scottish Dental Clinical Effectiveness Programme (SDCP). Drug prescribing for dentistry. https://www.sdcep.org.uk/published-guidance/drug-prescribing/ (accessed 25 February 2024).

RESOURCES FOR DENTAL PATIENTS

ADA (American Dental Association). MouthHealthy article: "Will antibiotics help treat my dental pain?" https://www.mouthhealthy.org/all-topics-a-z/antibiotics-for-pain-and-swelling/ (accessed 25 February 2024).

REFERENCES

1. Cope, A.L., Francis, N., Wood, F., and Chestnutt, I.G. (2018). Systemic antibiotics for symptomatic apical periodontitis and acute apical abscess in adults. *Cochrane Database of Systematic Reviews* 2018: CD010136.

2. Lockhart, P.B., Tampi, M.P., Abt, E. et al. (2019). Evidence-based clinical practice guideline on antibiotic use for the urgent management of pulpal- and periapical-related dental pain and intraoral swelling: a report from the American Dental Association. *The Journal of the American Dental Association* 150 (11): 906–921.

3. Ali, K., Venkatasami, N., Zahra, D. et al. (2021). Evaluation of sepsis teaching for medical and dental students at a British University. *European Journal of Dental Education* 26: 296–301.

4. Ali, K., Mccarthy, A., Robbins, J. et al. (2014). Management of impacted wisdom teeth: teaching of undergraduate students in UK dental schools. *European Journal of Dental Education* 18 (3): 135–141.

5. Caruso, S.R., Yamaguchi, E., and Portnof, J.E. (2022). Update on antimicrobial therapy in management of acute odontogenic infection in oral and maxillofacial surgery. *Oral and Maxillofacial Surgery Clinics of North America* 34: 169–177.

6. The UK Sepsis Trust (2022). About Sepsis. https://sepsistrust.org/about/about-sepsis/ (accessed September 2023).

7. Dave, M., Barry, S., Coulthard, P. et al. (2021). An evaluation of sepsis in dentistry. *British Dental Journal* 230 (6): 351–357.

Use of Antibiotics in Periodontitis

CHAPTER 5

Ewen McColl[1] and Kamran Ali[2]

[1] *Plymouth University, Faculty of Health (Medicine, Dentistry, and Human Sciences), Department of Clinical Dentistry, Plymouth, UK*
[2] *Qatar University, QU Health, College of Dental Medicine, Doha, Qatar*

5.1 INTRODUCTION

Diverse communities of oral microbiome are essential for periodontal health. However bacterial dysbiosis may occur, resulting in the predominance of certain pathogenic strains that induce the inflammatory host response and symptoms associated with periodontitis and clinical sequelae that may follow. Periodontal pathogens, known as red complex bacteria, are more strongly associated with periodontitis and loss of clinical attachment[1]. These red complex bacteria, may become more prevalent during late stages of biofilm development resulting in a dysbiosis and possible damage to the periodontium. Patient home maintenance and Professional Mechanical Plaque removal (PMPR) are key to reversing this dysbiosis. Contrary to the previous belief that adjunctive systemic antibiotics in severe cases of disease may contribute to reversing this dysbiosis, the risks associated with antibiotic resistance are recognised globally and widespread use of antibiotics can lead to disruption of the oral microbiome and may not offer substantial benefits in resolution of periodontal disease[2].

In 2017, a new classification system was developed in the World Workshop on the Classification of Periodontal and Peri-Implant Diseases and Conditions[3, 4]. The new periodontal classification led to a shift in the way clinicians classify and diagnose periodontal diseases. This staging and grading of disease led to a move away from classifying disease as chronic or aggressive and with that a change in the way antibiotics were prescribed. In particular, antibiotics had often been used as adjunct to non-surgical periodontal therapy in the management of aggressive periodontitis as it was classified then, and this is no longer the case. This change in emphasis on understanding a continuum of disease means that antibiotics should never be prescribed based on a specific disease classification but prescribed sparingly in line with regularly updated professional guidelines.

Whilst antibiotics may have a role to play in the more acute periodontal conditions, – this should in general only be the case if the patient is pyrexic, there is a risk of a spreading infection and prior to prescribing – local drainage of pus should be attempted. This is particularly the case in periodontal abscesses where the old adage 'if there's pus about, let it out' is more relevant than ever.

There are various modes of delivery of antibiotics in periodontal disease are described in the following section.

5.2 ROLE OF SYSTEMIC ANTIBIOTICS IN PERIODONTAL DISEASE

Whilst systemic antibiotics were commonly prescribed for aggressive periodontitis, the doses were often very high and likely to contribute to antibiotic resistance. Early studies by van Winkelhoff

---

Clinical Dental Pharmacology, First Edition. Edited by Kamran Ali.
© 2024 John Wiley & Sons Ltd. Published 2024 by John Wiley & Sons Ltd.

reported use of amoxicillin and metronidazole which had positive results in aggressive periodontitis cases but were poorly tolerated by patients and had an elevated risk of antibiotic resistance[5]. The advantage of systemic antibiotics was that high levels were achieved in the bloodstream systemically, but this was not so certain in periodontal pockets, and of course consistent doses were reliant on patient compliance.

Concerns about antibiotic resistance are now widespread, and use is very much determined by systemic symptoms such as pyrexia and spreading infection[6]. Whilst antibiotics may be used in managing severe cases of periodontitis in young patients, this would be far rarer than previously, and for general dental practitioners referral to a Specialist Periodontist would be indicated. It is crucial to follow professional guidelines on antibiotic prescribing[7].

On referral to a specialist where patients have severe disease at an early age (Stage III, IV periodontitis Grade C in patients aged <35–45 years), antibiotics may be considered. As always optimising oral hygiene measures by patients and PMPR are crucial to success and prescription of antibiotics should never be done in isolation. Where antibiotics are to be used, the biofilm should be disturbed using PMPR and antibiotic usage commenced on the same day as this extensive PMPR is completed. There is some evidence of effectiveness of completing the PMPR in one day. However, if patient tolerance does not allow this, the PMPR should be completed, ideally within a week.

A range of systematic reviews have demonstrated that use of systemic antimicrobials as an adjunct to PMPR which can result in greater PD reductions and gains in CAL compared to just root surface debridement (RSD) alone[8, 9]. In many of these studies, amoxicillin is used conjunctively with metronidazole. The doses are high, and systemic complications such as nausea and vomiting likely occur. This must also be very carefully considered alongside the risk of antibiotic resistance more generally at a population level, so specialist consideration of antibiotic use must be supported with careful operative management of the patient's condition.

5.3 ROLE OF LOCAL DELIVERY ANTIBIOTICS IN PERIODONTAL DISEASE

Local delivery antibiotics surmount the inconsistencies of antibiotic levels in periodontal pockets by applying the antibiotic directly and are generally well tolerated by patients. Whilst commercial availability may vary by country, the most popular local delivery antibiotics used for the treatment of periodontitis include:

- 25% Metronidazole gel (Elyzol®)

- 2% Minocycline presented in bio-resorbable spheres (Arestin®)

- 2% Minocycline gel (Dentomycin®)

Elyzol® consists of an oil-based metronidazole 25% dental gel, which consists of glyceryl mono-oleate and triglyceride (sesame oil). The gel is placed subgingivally with a syringe and a blunt cannula, and the manufacturer suggests the metronidazole is released in an exponential pattern compatible with sustained drug delivery.

Arestin® consists of 2% minocycline encapsulated into bio-resorbable microspheres in a gel carrier. The gingival crevicular fluid hydrolyses the polymer and releases minocycline with associated antibacterial affect.

In the case of minocycline gels (Dentomycin®) due to the gel being washed out by gingival crevicular fluid and blood flow, application is repeated fortnightly on 3 occasions. Evidence for improvements in clinical parameters is inconsistent and when one considers cost benefit, then this has to be discussed with the patient at the time of consent (Figure 5.1)[10].

Clinically, the evidence appears to suggest that local delivery antimicrobials such as minocycline and metronidazole are best used in controlling localised disease in otherwise stable

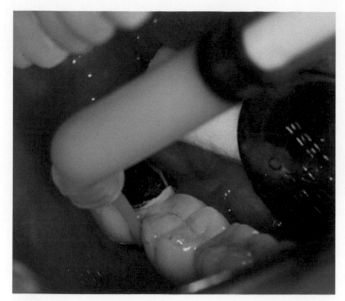

FIGURE 5.1 Application of Dentomycin® to periodontal pocket

patients. This means specific sites can be targeted. Similarly in maintenance patients with localised nonresponding or recurring sites, local delivery antibiotics may be helpful.

5.4 USE OF LOW DOSE (SUB-ANTIMICROBIAL) ANTIMICROBIALS

Doxycycline used in sub-antimicrobial doses has been suggested for use in the management of periodontal diseases. Rather than affecting the oral microbiome, the suggested mode of action is due to the anticollagenase effect of the doxycycline.

Clinical trials included in a systematic review which analysed 3 trials using sub-antimicrobial doses of doxycycline for 3 months compared to RSD alone have revealed limited improvements in clinical parameters (0.9 mm extra reduction in pocket depth)[11]. Further systematic reviews have revealed limited improvements in clinical parameters (Gain in Clinical Attachment levels of 0.15–0.56 mm). Given the small gains and risks in taking any systemic medicine, not least an antimicrobial, it is doubtful in a risk benefit analysis that this route will be indicated in managing periodontitis patients, particularly given the long-term need to take this medicine, i.e., 3 months as recommended by the manufacturer.

5.5 NECROTISING PERIODONTAL DISEASES

In the previous 1999 classification, necrotising periodontal diseases (NPD) were classified as 'necrotising ulcerative gingivitis' and 'necrotising ulcerative periodontitis'. In the 2017 classification system, NPDs are defined as: necrotising gingivitis (NG), necrotising periodontitis (NP), necrotising stomatitis (NS), and Noma. Clinically, it can be challenging to differentiate between NG and NP. Studies suggest that NG, NP, NS, and Noma are various stages of the same disease as they share clinical characteristics and, to some extent, treatment[12].

The management principles of different forms of NPDs are discussed in the following section.

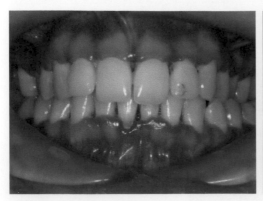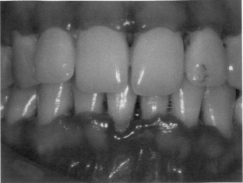

FIGURE 5.2 Presentation of necrotising periodontal disease

5.5.1 NECROTISING GINGIVITIS, NECROTISING PERIODONTITIS

- Determine a definitive diagnosis.

- Address underlying risk factors:

- *Local*: poor oral hygiene, pre-existing gingivitis/periodontitis:
  - *Systemic*: Smoking, stress, early age, malnutrition, and immunosuppression (e.g., AIDS, HIV-positive, leukaemia, cyclic neutropenia); may require consultation with a medical physician.

- *Supportive measures*:
  - Advice and demonstrations to improve oral hygiene,
  - Analgesics,
  - Improve fluid intake, and
  - Rest.

- *Management of acute phase*:
  - Gentle debridement using a hand scaler or ultrasonic device under local anaesthesia,

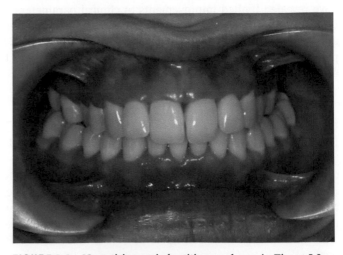

FIGURE 5.3 Necrotising periodontitis case shown in Figure 5.2 after treatment

- Mouthwashes such as saline rinses in hot water; 6% hydrogen peroxide mouthwash or 0.2% chlorhexidine,
- Pain control with oral paracetamol,
- *Antibiotics*: In instances where the patient has systemic features such as fever, malaise, lymphadenopathy, systemic antibiotics may be indicated.
  - Metronidazole is selected as the first-line antibiotic treatment, effective against anaerobes, including the fusospirochaetal anaerobes associated with this disease. The recommended dose of metronidazole (tablets) in adults is 400 mg 8 hourly for 3–5 days. For patients aged 10–17 years, the dose is halved, i.e., 200 mg 8 hourly.
  - If a patient is unable to take metronidazole (for instance, due to alcohol intake or allergies), consider amoxicillin capsules 500 mg 8 hourly in adults and 250 mg 8 hourly in 12–17-year-old patients.
- *Maintenance phase*:
  - Regular follow-up to maintain and reinforce oral hygiene. The loss of papillary architecture may mean oral hygiene regimes have to be tailored accordingly and appropriate sizing of interdental brushes.
  - Review risk factors will be essential in this maintenance phase.

5.5.2 NECROTISING STOMATITIS

NS is a further progression of the disease with risk factors as discussed previously. NS as with the other diseases is painful, and when the gingival architecture is so severely compromised, this can lead to exposure of the underlying alveolar bone which can also necrose. The clinical presentation is similar to the other NPDs with a higher likelihood of pyrexia and cervical lymphadenopathy, with patients often feeling systemically unwell. Management is generally similar to NPD. Severe cases may require referral to specialists based in a hospital setting.

5.5.3 NOMA

The World Health Organization describe Noma as 'Noma (from Greek: to "devour") is a necrotising destructive disease with superadded putrefaction affecting the mouth and the face'. This disease is characterised by necrotising fasciitis, osteonecrosis and myonecrosis, that leads to severe facial disfigurement and disability[13]. Figure 5.3 indicates presentation of the disease as it affects

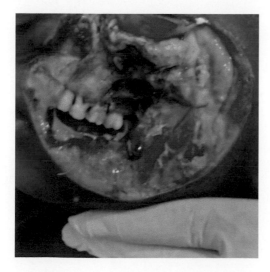

FIGURE 5.4 Oral soft tissue destruction in Noma

the circumoral soft tissue, in many cases affecting the whole of the face. Whilst metronidazole is extremely effective in the initial stages, established cases of Noma require aggressive management under multidisciplinary medical and surgical team in specialist hospital settings (Figure 5.4).

5.6 SUMMARY

Whilst the use of antibiotics in periodontitis both systemically and locally has decreased since the adoption of the 2017 classification, there may be occasions when antibiotics are prescribed. For periodontitis, this should be done in conjunction with specialist input. Acute periodontal conditions with systemic involvement may justify a short course of antibiotics along with other measures as described earlier.

ACKNOWLEDGEMENTS

Figure 5.4 provided by Fatima Dantata/Adetula Ifeoluwa, Nigeria.

RESOURCES

RESOURCES FOR DENTAL PROFESSIONALS

Scottish Clinical Dental Effectiveness Programme (SDCEP). Prevention and Treatment of Periodontal Diseases in Primary Care, Second Edition (2024). https://www.sdcep.org.uk/published-guidance/periodontal-care/ (accessed 20 February 2024).

RESOURCES FOR DENTAL PATIENTS

Mayo Clinic. Periodontitis: symptoms, causes, diagnosis and treatment. https://www.mayoclinic .org/diseases-conditions/periodontitis/symptoms-causes/syc-20354473 (accessed 26 February 2024).

Cleveland Clinic. Periodontitis. https://my.clevelandclinic.org/health/diseases/16620-periodontitis (accessed 26 February 2024).

REFERENCES

1. Socransky, S.S., Haffajee, A.D., Cugini, M.A. et al. (1998). Microbial complexes in subgingival plaque. *Journal of Clinical Periodontology* 25 (2): 134–144.

2. Antimicrobial resistance. https://www.who .int/news-room/fact-sheets/detail/antimicrobial-resistance

3. Caton, J.G., Armitage, G., Berglundh, T. et al. (2018). A new classification scheme for periodontal and peri-implant diseases and conditions – introduction and key changes from the 1999 classification. *Journal of Clinical Periodontology* 89: 45.

4. Papapanou, P.N., Sanz, M., Buduneli, N. et al. (2018). Periodontitis: Consensus report of workgroup 2 of the 2017 World Workshop on the Classification of Periodontal and Peri-Implant Diseases and Conditions. *Journal of Periodontology* 89: S173–S182.

5. Van Winkelhoff, A.J., Herrera Gonzales, D., Winkel, E.G. et al. (2000). Antimicrobial resistance in the subgingival microflora in patients with adult periodontitis: a comparison between the Netherlands and Spain. *Journal of Clinical Periodontology* 27: 79–86.

6. The Lancet Global Health (2017). Fighting antimicrobial resistance on all fronts. *The Lancet Global Health* 5: e1161.

7. Drug prescribing | Scottish Dental Clinical Effectiveness Pr (2021). https://www.sdcep.org.uk/published-guidance/drug-prescribing/ (accessed 04 September 2023).

8. Keestra, J.A.J., Grosjean, I., Coucke, W. et al. (2015). Non-surgical periodontal therapy with systemic antibiotics in patients with untreated chronic periodontitis: a systematic review and meta-analysis. *Journal of Periodontal Research* 50: 294–314.

9. Herrera, D., Sanz, M., Jepsen, S. et al. (2002). A systematic review on the effect of systemic antimicrobials as an adjunct to scaling and root planing in periodontitis patients. *Journal of Clinical Periodontology* 29: 136–159.

10. Herrera, D., Matesanz, P., Martín, C. et al. (2020). Adjunctive effect of locally delivered antimicrobials in periodontitis therapy: a systematic review and meta-analysis. *Journal of Clinical Periodontology* 47: 239–256.

11. Sgolastra, F., Petrucci, A., Gatto, R. et al. (2011). Long-term efficacy of subantimicrobial-dose doxycycline as an adjunctive treatment to scaling and root planing: a systematic review and meta-analysis. *Journal of Periodontology* 82 (11): 1570–1581.

12. Ogunleye, R., Ukoha, O., Nasterska, W. et al. (2022). Necrotising periodontal diseases: an update on classification and management. *British Dental Journal* 233 (10): 855–858.

13. Farley, E., Mehta, U., Leila Srour, M., and Lenglet, A. (2021). Noma (cancrumoris): a scoping literature review of a neglected disease (1843 to 2021). *PLoS Neglected Tropical Diseases* 15 (12): e0009844.

CHAPTER 6

Antibiotic Prophylaxis Against Infective Endocarditis in Dentistry

Kamran Ali

Qatar University, QU Health, College of Dental Medicine, Doha, Qatar

6.1 INTRODUCTION

Infective endocarditis (IE) is a potentially life-threatening infection of the inner lining of the heart (endocardium) and often involves the heart valves. Invasive dental procedures may result in a transient bacteraemia which may lead to IE. The most recognised symptoms of IE are summarised as follows:

- An elevated temperature (fever) of 38 °C or above

- Sweats or chills, especially at night

- Breathlessness, especially during physical activity

- Weight loss

- Tiredness (fatigue)

- Muscle, joint, or back pain (unrelated to recent physical activity)

All patients at increased risk of IE should be advised to contact their medical physician or local hospital as soon as possible if they notice any of the aforementioned symptoms, particularly if they occur together as a flu-like illness. Untreated IE is associated with several cardiac complications and carries an elevated risk of morbidity and mortality.

Previously, sporadic high-grade bacteraemia (α haemolytic *Streptococcus viridans*) caused by invasive dental procedures was considered to be the main risk factor for IE of oral origin, with consequent widespread use of antibiotic prophylaxis for all patients considered to be at risk. However, the current guidelines advise against routine use of antibiotic prophylaxis due to several reasons:

- There is lack of clarity regarding the risk of bacteraemia following dental procedures[1].

- Cumulative, low-grade bacteraemia, triggered by normal daily activities such as tooth brushing, flossing, and chewing, are of greater significance. Prevention of IE in patients at risk requires maintenance of good oral and skin hygiene, and regular professional dental care.

- The evidence base for the efficacy of antibiotic prophylaxis for endocarditis is weak and views on the risk–benefit analysis have shifted in recent years, with moves to reduce the utilisation of antibiotic prophylaxis[2].

Therefore, the use of antibiotics should be considered carefully due to their side effects and risk of adverse reactions, development of antibiotic resistance, and cost.

Clinical Dental Pharmacology, First Edition. Edited by Kamran Ali.
© 2024 John Wiley & Sons Ltd. Published 2024 by John Wiley & Sons Ltd.

Table 6.1   Conditions Associated with High Risk of Developing Infective Endocarditis[a]

- Prosthetic heart valves, including a transcatheter valve and homograft.
- Cardiac valve repair with any prosthetic material.
- Previous episode of IE.
- Cardiac transplant with valve regurgitation due to structural valvular abnormalities.
- Unrepaired cyanotic congenital heart disease (CHD), including palliative shunts or conduits.
- Repaired CHD repaired with a prosthetic material, whether placed surgically or by percutaneous techniques, up to 6 months after the procedure or lifelong in the presence of a residual shunt or valvular regurgitation.

[a] Patients with cardiac stents or pacemakers are not considered to be at an increased risk of IE, and antibiotic prophylaxis is not required in such patients.

6.2 INDICATIONS FOR ANTIBIOTIC PROPHYLAXIS

National and regional guidelines on antibiotic prophylaxis against IE have been produced by several professional organisations globally, and dentists are advised to follow relevant guidelines applicable in their country. For countries, where national guidelines are not available, dentists are signposted to professional guidelines in the United Kingdom and United States which are broadly similar. Although several cardiac conditions may theoretically increase the risk of endocarditis, currently antibiotic prophylaxis is recommended primarily for patients who are at the highest risk of developing endocarditis following invasive dental procedure (Table 6.1). Re-assessment of the decision on antibiotic prophylaxis is required if there is a change in the patient's medical history.

Dentists usually do not have access to the full cardiac history of their patients and whenever, possible, a dentist must consult with the patient's cardiologist/cardiac surgeon for advice.

6.3 DENTAL PROCEDURES

In patients considered to be at risk (Table 6.1), prophylaxis is recommended for all invasive dental procedures that involve manipulation of gingival tissue or the periapical region of the teeth, or perforation of the oral mucosa as summarised in Table 6.2.

Table 6.2   Classification of Dental Procedures[3]

Invasive dental procedures	Non-invasive dental procedures
- Placement of sub-gingival rubber dam clamps/matrix bands - Sub-gingival restorations including fixed prosthodontics. - Endodontic treatment before apical seal has been established. - Preformed metal crowns - Full periodontal examinations (including pocket charting) - Root surface instrumentation/sub-gingival scaling - Incision and drainage of abscess - Dental extractions - Oral/periodontal surgery involving elevation mucoperiosteal mucogingival flaps. - Placement of dental implants, including temporary anchorage devices and mini-implants - Uncovering implant sub-structures	- Infiltration or block local anaesthetic injections in non-infected soft tissues. - BPE screening - Supra-gingival restorations - Supra-gingival scale and polish - Supra-gingival orthodontic bands and separators - Removal of sutures - Radiographs - Placement or adjustment of orthodontic or removable prosthodontic appliances

BPE, basic periodontal examination.
Antibiotic prophylaxis is not recommended following exfoliation of primary teeth or trauma to the lips or oral mucosa.

Table 6.3 Antibiotic Regimens for a Dental Procedure Regimen, United Kingdom

Agent	Dose in adults	Dose in children
Single oral dose 60 minutes before procedure		
First choice: Amoxicillin	3 g Oral powder sachet	6 months–17 years: 50 mg/kg; maximum dose 3 g Appropriate dose may be administered using either amoxicillin oral suspension 250 mg/5 mL or 3-g oral powder sachet.
Second choice: Clindamycin	600 mg 2 × 300 mg capsules with water	6 months–17 years: 20 mg/kg; maximum dose 600 mg Accurate dose may be administered using either clindamycin capsules 300 mg or clindamycin oral suspension/syrup 75 mg/5 mL, as appropriate.
Third choice: Azithromycin	500 mg Oral suspension 200 mg/5 mL; administer 12.5 mL	6–11 years: 12 mg/kg; maximum dose 500 mg 12–17 years: 500 mg Accurate dose may be administered using azithromycin oral suspension 200 mg/5 mL
Single intravenous dose at induction (unable to take oral medication or treatment under GA)		
Amoxicillin	1 g just before the procedure or at induction of anaesthesia	6 months–17 years: 50 mg/kg; maximum dose 1 g
Clindamycin	300 mg just before the procedure or at induction of anaesthesia	6 months–17 years: 20 mg/kg; maximum dose 300 mg

Source: Refs.3, 4.

Table 6.4 Antibiotic Regimens for a Dental Procedure, United States: Single Dose 30–60 minutes Before Procedure[5]

Situation	Agent	Adults	Children
Oral	Amoxicillin	2 g	50 mg/kg
Unable to take oral medication	Ampicillin Or	2 g IM or IV	50 mg/kg IM or IV
	Cefazolin Or Ceftriaxone	1 g IM or IV	50 mg/kg IM or IV
Allergic to penicillin or ampicillin – oral	Cephalexin[a,b]	2 g	50 mg/kg
	Or Azithromycin Or Clarithromycin	500 mg	15 mg/kg
	or Doxycycline	100 mg	<45 kg, 2.2 mg/kg >45 kg, 100 mg
Allergic to penicillin or ampicillin and unable to take oral medication	Cefazolin or Ceftriaxone[b]	1 g IM or IV	50 mg/kg IM or IV

Clindamycin is no longer recommended for antibiotic prophylaxis for a dental procedure.

IM, intramuscular; IV, intravenous.

[a] Or other first- or second-generation oral cephalosporin in equivalent adult or paediatric dosing.

[b] Cephalosporins should not be used in an individual with a history of anaphylaxis, angioedema, or urticarial with penicillin or ampicillin.

6.4 ANTIBIOTIC REGIMENS

There are some differences in antibiotic dose and timing in different countries. Antibiotic regimens in the United Kingdom (Table 6.3) and United States (Table 6.4) are discussed in this section. However, readers are advised to follow guidelines in their own country or if these are unavailable, they may choose one of the following antibiotic regimens. In any case, dentists must consider side effects, contra-indications and cautions for the individual antibiotic (see Chapter 3). Patients should be consented appropriately for antibiotic prophylaxis, and contemporaneous clinical records must be maintained. Also, patients should be followed up for the identification of symptoms suggestive of IE to facilitate prompt referral and management.

6.5 SUMMARY

Dentists should always follow national guidelines on antibiotic prophylaxis against bacterial endocarditis prior to invasive dental procedures. Although antibiotic cover is generally reserved for patients with high-risk cardiac conditions, it is best to provide adequate information to the patients to help them make an informed consent. Whenever there are any doubts regarding the need for antibiotic prophylaxis prior to dental procedures, it may be appropriate to seek advice from the patient's cardiologist. All discussions with the patient or their caregivers must be documented comprehensively.

RESOURCES

RESOURCES FOR DENTAL PROFESSIONALS

American Dental Association (ADA). Antibiotic prophylaxis prior to dental procedures. https://www.ada.org/resources/ada-library/oral-health-topics/antibiotic-prophylaxis (accessed February 2024).

Scottish Dental Clinical Excellence Programme (SDCEP). Implementation advice for National Institute for Health and Care Excellence (NICE) Clinical Guideline 64 prophylaxis against infective endocarditis, https://www.sdcep.org.uk/published-guidance/antibiotic-prophylaxis/ (accessed February 2024).

Australian Dental Association (ADA). Prevention of endocarditis: Dental procedures (2014). https://ada.org.au/getmedia/653d5907-1e3a-4f50-90c6-577ddf79e6cd/Therapeutic-Guidelines-Limited_Guidelines_Prevention-of-Endocarditis.pdf (accessed February 2024).

RESOURCES FOR DENTAL PATIENTS

Cleveland Clinic. Endocarditis. https://my.clevelandclinic.org/health/diseases/16957-endocarditis (accessed February 2024).

REFERENCES

1. Navarro, B.G., Salas, E.J., Devesa, A.E. et al. (2017). Bacteremia associated with oral surgery: a review. *The Journal of Evidence-Based Dental Practice* 17 (3): 190–204.

2. Rutherford, S.J., Glenny, A.M., Roberts, G. et al. (2022). Antibiotic prophylaxis for preventing bacterial endocarditis following dental procedures. *Cochrane Database of Systematic Reviews* (5): CD003813.

3. Antibiotic prophylaxis | Scottish Dental Clinical Effectiven. https://www.sdcep.org.uk/published-guidance/antibiotic-prophylaxis/ (accessed 23 February 2024).

4. National Institute for Health and Care Excellence (2015). *Prophylaxis Against Infective Endocarditis*. National Institute for Health and Care Excellence.

5. Wilson, W.R., Gewitz, M., Lockhart, P.B. et al. (2021). Prevention of viridans group streptococcal infective endocarditis: a scientific statement from the American Heart Association. *Circulation* 143 (20): e963–e978.

Antimicrobial Resistance CHAPTER 7

Susu M. Zughaier and Kamran Ali

Qatar University, QU Health, College of Dental Medicine, Doha, Qatar

7.1 INTRODUCTION

Antibiotic era dawned in 1928 with the discovery of penicillin. The success of penicillin led to a search for other antibacterial molecules and heralded a golden age of antibiotic discovery, which continued from the 1940s to the 1970s. This changed the medical and public expectations and revolutionised the practice of medicine. However, with time, antimicrobial resistance (AMR) has increased in magnitude progressively. Although AMR can be associated with any type of antimicrobial agent, it is primarily contributed by antibiotics due to their widespread use. AMR is a global health problem, and the World Health Organization (WHO) has declared AMR as one of the top 10 global public health threats facing humanity[1]. AMR contributes significantly to morbidity and mortality especially in hospitalised patients and can translates into a marked cost to the economy. An estimated 4.59 million deaths have been reported to be associated with bacterial AMR in 2019 making it is one of the leading causes of death globally[2]. Contemporary medicine must continue to develop and sustain options for combating microbial infections effectively failing which infections associated with surgical procedures and cancer chemotherapy would become a major threat and may even render these interventions unfeasible.

Dentists prescribe a variety of antimicrobials for prophylactic and therapeutic purposes[3]. However, apart from a few countries, up-to-date clinical guidelines on antimicrobials are not used consistently by dentists leading to risks of inappropriate and over-prescription of antimicrobials to dental patients. Limited longitudinal data are available on antimicrobial prescriptions by dentists to quantify the contribution of dental prescriptions to AMR. A study on dental prescriptions by dentists in England showed that dental prescriptions accounted for 10.8% of all oral antibiotic prescribing, 18.4% of amoxicillin and 57.0% of metronidazole prescribing in primary care settings[4]. Apparently, the antibiotic prescriptions by dentists in developed countries appear to show a decline, but further improvements are warranted.

7.2 COMMON DRIVERS OF ANTIBIOTIC RESISTANCE

A number of factors may contribute to increase in antibiotic-resistant microorganisms in domestic, healthcare and industrial settings[1]. The main causes include the following:

i. *Overuse of antibiotics*
   Overuse and misuse of antibiotics are the primary drivers of antibiotic resistance. When antibiotics are overused or used inappropriately, bacteria have more opportunities to develop resistance to them.

ii. *Incomplete treatment*
   Failure to complete a full course of antibiotic treatment can also contribute to antibiotic resistance. When bacteria are exposed to antibiotics for a short period of time, they may not be completely eradicated, allowing them to continue reproducing and developing resistance.

Clinical Dental Pharmacology, First Edition. Edited by Kamran Ali.
© 2024 John Wiley & Sons Ltd. Published 2024 by John Wiley & Sons Ltd.

iii. *Agricultural use of antibiotics*

Antibiotics are often used in agriculture to prevent and treat disease in livestock. This can contribute to antibiotic resistance, as bacteria in animals can develop resistance and spread to humans through consumption of contaminated meat.

iv. *Poor infection control in healthcare settings*

Inadequate infection control practices can also contribute to the spread of antibiotic-resistant bacteria. For example, failure to properly clean and disinfect surfaces in healthcare settings can allow bacteria to spread and potentially develop resistance.

v. *Poor hygiene and sanitation in community settings*

Poor hygiene, lack of access to clean water and inadequate sanitation facilities in community settings also increase the risk of antibiotic-resistant microorganism in the environment.

vi. *Lack of new antibiotics*

There has been a decline in the development of new antibiotics in recent years, which has made it more difficult to treat infections caused by antibiotic-resistant bacteria. This decline was mainly driven by the emergence of AMR to newly developed antibiotics and the associated economic burden.

7.3 MECHANISMS OF ANTIBIOTIC RESISTANCE

Several key mechanisms are involved in the development of antibiotic resistance that allow bacteria to survive and proliferate in the presence of antibiotics as depicted in Figure 7.1.

The mechanisms involved in AMR resistance with relevant examples are summarised in Table 7.1.

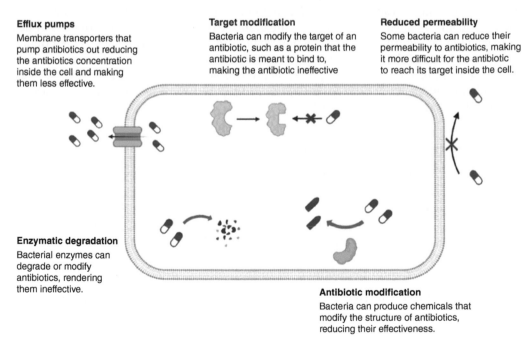

Efflux pumps

Membrane transporters that pump antibiotics out reducing the antibiotics concentration inside the cell and making them less effective.

Target modification

Bacteria can modify the target of an antibiotic, such as a protein that the antibiotic is meant to bind to, making the antibiotic ineffective

Reduced permeability

Some bacteria can reduce their permeability to antibiotics, making it more difficult for the antibiotic to reach its target inside the cell.

Enzymatic degradation

Bacterial enzymes can degrade or modify antibiotics, rendering them ineffective.

Antibiotic modification

Bacteria can produce chemicals that modify the structure of antibiotics, reducing their effectiveness.

FIGURE 7.1 Schematic illustration of common mechanisms responsible for antimicrobial resistance. Source: Image created in http://BioRender.com

Table 7.1 Bacterial Mechanisms of Developing Resistance to Antibiotics

Bacterial mechanism	Examples
Enzymatic degradation Bacterial enzymes can degrade or modify antibiotics, rendering them ineffective.	*Staphylococcus aureus* producing β-lactamases that can degrade penicillin antibiotics.
Efflux pumps Membrane transporters that pump antibiotics out of the bacterial cell, reducing the concentration of antibiotics inside the cell and making them less effective.	*Pseudomonas aeruginosa* that pumps out fluoroquinolone antibiotics, a class of antibiotics used to treat urinary tract infections and other bacterial infections. *Escherichia coli* that pumps out tetracycline antibiotics, a class of antibiotics used to treat respiratory and urinary tract infections.
Target modification Bacteria can modify the target of an antibiotic, such as a protein that the antibiotic is meant to bind to, making the antibiotic ineffective	Methicillin-resistant *Staphylococcus aureus* (MRSA) produces a modified penicillin-binding protein that has reduced affinity for ß-lactam antibiotics, making them ineffective. Modification of targets of macrolide antibiotics *Streptococcus pneumoniae*
Reduced permeability Some bacteria can reduce their permeability to antibiotics, making it more difficult for the antibiotic to enter the cell and reach its target.	*Mycobacterium tuberculosis* that has a thick, waxy cell wall that reduces the penetration of antibiotics, making it difficult to treat tuberculosis infections. *E. coli* harbouring mcr-1 plasmid that encodes phosphoethanolamine transferase enzyme confers resistance to colistin.
Antibiotic modification Bacteria can produce chemicals that modify the structure of antibiotics, reducing their effectiveness.	*Streptomyces* spp. produce enzymes that modify the structure of erythromycin *Enterococcus faecalis* produces a protein that can modify and inactivate aminoglycosides
Biofilm formation Bacteria can form biofilms encased in a protective matrix which reduce the penetration of the antibiotic into the biofilm	*Pseudomonas aeruginosa* forms biofilms in the lungs of cystic fibrosis *Staphylococcus epidermidis* forms biofilms on medical devices, such as catheters and prosthetic joints

7.4 TACKLING ANTIBIOTIC RESISTANCE

7.4.1 GENERAL MEASURES

1. Improvements in infection prevention and control practices.

2. Optimisation of prescribing practice.

3. Improvements in professional education, training and public engagement.

4. Development of new drugs, treatments and diagnostics.

5. Better collection, access and use of surveillance data.

6. Prioritisation of AMR research through international collaboration.

7.4.2 MEASURES IN DENTAL SETTINGS

- Patient education to emphasise the following:
  - Maintenance of meticulous oral hygiene remains the most fundamental measure to prevent dental disease.
  - Regular professional dental care for early recognition and management of dental disease
  - Antibiotics are not always the best option to treat dental pain and infection.
  - Antibiotics do not compensate for suboptimal operative management of dental disease.
  - Advise patients to complete the course of antibiotics.
  - Dispose of unused antibiotics appropriately.
  - Resist any temptation to self-medicate using left over antibiotics.
- Prescribe antibiotics only when necessary (Chapter 4).
- Do not prescribe antibiotics solely on patient's request.
- Develop antibiotic stewardship in clinical dental practice settings.
- Undertake regular audit of antibiotic prescriptions.

7.5 SUMMARY

AMR is a serious global issue, compounded by the limited progress in the development of new antibiotics. The main category of antimicrobials prescribed by dentists is antibiotics, while antifungal and antiviral medications are prescribed less frequently in clinical dental settings. To combat this issue, it is imperative that antibiotic prescriptions are restricted to clinical situations where they are absolutely essential.

It is suggested that dental professionals demonstrate a commitment to prevent inappropriate use of antibiotics in their own settings to minimise AMR. Any healthcare professional can make a pledge to become an antibiotic guardian at https://antibioticguardian.com. The site provides useful resources on prevention on antibiotic resistance including materials for patient education. Dentists are encouraged to actively educate their patients on the risks of AMR. A fundamental message which needs to reiterated is that antibiotics are not a suitable treatment option for most dental problems, and their use must be restricted to specific clinical situations.

Dentists may develop patient information leaflets, posters and other forms of educational materials which may be shared with the patients, their caregivers and the public at large. Disseminating risks of antibiotic resistance to both colleagues and patients can help to raise awareness of the importance of using antibiotics responsibly and encourage more judicious use of these drugs.

ACKNOWLEDGEMENTS

Figure 7.1 provided by Ms Maryam Hassiba, Qatar University.

RESOURCES

RESOURCES FOR DENTAL PROFESSIONALS

Antibiotic Guardian. Become an antibiotic guardian. https://antibioticguardian.com (accessed February 2024).

World Health Organisation (WHO). Antibiotic resistance. https://www.who.int/news-room/fact-sheets/detail/antibiotic-resistance (accessed February 2024).

RESOURCES FOR DENTAL PATIENTS

European Centre for Disease Prevention and Control. Factsheet for the general public – Antimicrobial resistance. https://www.ecdc.europa.eu/en/antimicrobial-resistance/facts/factsheets/general-public (accessed February 2024).

World Health Organization (WHO). Antibiotic resistance. https://www.who.int/news-room/fact-sheets/detail/antibiotic-resistance (accessed February 2024).

REFERENCES

1. World Health Organisation (WHO) (2023). Antimicrobial resistance. https://www.who.int/news-room/fact-sheets/detail/antimicrobial-resistance (accessed 25 February 2024).

2. Murray, C.J., Ikuta, K.S., Sharara, F. et al. (2022). Global burden of bacterial antimicrobial resistance in 2019: a systematic analysis. *The Lancet* 399 (10325): 629–655.

3. Kariyawasam, R.M., Julien, D.A., Jelinski, D.C. et al. (2022). Antimicrobial resistance (AMR) in COVID-19 patients: a systematic review and meta-analysis (November 2019–June 2021). *Antimicrobial Resistance and Infection Control* 11 (1): 45.

4. Thornhill, M.H., Dayer, M.J., Durkin, M.J. et al. (2019). Oral antibiotic prescribing by NHS dentists in England 2010–2017. *British Dental Journal* 227 (12): 1044–1050.

CHAPTER 8 | Antiviral Medications

Sadeq Ali Al-Maweri and Kamran Ali

Qatar University, QU Health, College of Dental Medicine, Doha, Qatar

8.1 INTRODUCTION

Viral infections of orofacial soft tissues are well recognised and may be associated with significant discomfort and complications.[1] Although many viral infections can involve the orofacial region, infections caused by the herpes group viruses are the most common.[2] Also known as Herpesviridae, herpes viruses comprise a large group of DNA viruses (over 130 are known so far) that cause various infections in animals and humans.[3, 4] Human infections are associated with eight types of human herpes virus (HHV).[4] HHVs are neurotropic, i.e., they have the ability to reside within the nerves of the host in a latent form and cause recurrent infections. HHV group includes the following viruses:

- *HHV-1 Herpes simplex virus-1 (HSV-1)*: Predominantly causes oral herpes; also associated with genital herpes.

- *HHV-1 Herpes simplex virus-2 (HSV-2)*: Predominantly causes genital herpes; also associated with oral herpes due to cross-contamination following oro-genital contact.

    Primary oral herpes usually affects children and presents as herpetic gingivostomatitis characterised by vesicular eruptions which rupture to leave painful ulcerations on the oral mucosa, accompanied by erythematous marginal gingivitis with bleeding. In adults, primary herpes presents as pharyngotonsillitis. Recurrent herpes most commonly manifests as herpetic labialis (*cold sores* on lips), and *herpetic whitlow* on skin of fingers. Chronic oral herpes may also be associated with aphthous ulcers, erythema multiforme and oral carcinomas.

- *HV-3 Varicella zoster*: Primary infection causes chicken pox; reactivation of virus causes shingles. Clinically shingles presents with unilateral involvement of skin characterised by clusters of vesicles followed by extremely painful ulcerations in the distribution of one of the branches of the trigeminal nerve, as shown in Figure 8.1. Shingles may also be complicated by post-herpetic neuralgia (Chapter 2) and Ramsay Hunt syndrome (facial paralysis, hearing defects and vertigo).

- *HHV-4 Epstein-Bar Virus (EBV)*: Causes infectious mononucleosis characterised by fever, malaise, anorexia and cervical lymphadenopathy. This presentation is often referred to as *glandular fever* and may also be seen in infection with HHV-4, HHV-6, HIV, *Toxoplasma gondii* (toxoplasmosis), Brucella (brucellosis) and also in patients with leukaemia. Other manifestations of EBV infection include hairy leukoplasia (immunocompromised patients), Burkitt's lymphoma, nasopharyngeal carcinoma and some forms of Hodgkin's lymphoma

- *HHV-5 Cytomegalovirus (CMV)*: CMV infection also causes glandular fever, similar to EBV.

- *HHV-6 Roseolovirus*: HHV-6 infection manifests with maculopapular skin rashes in infants and children (Exanthema subitem). HHV-6 has also been associated with multiple sclerosis (see Chapter 2).

Clinical Dental Pharmacology, First Edition. Edited by Kamran Ali.
© 2024 John Wiley & Sons Ltd. Published 2024 by John Wiley & Sons Ltd.

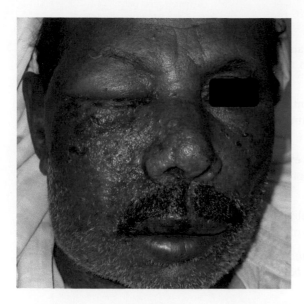

FIGURE 8.1   Herpes zoster infection of the face in the distribution of the right infra-orbital branch of the trigeminal nerve

- *HHV-7*: Similar manifestations as HHV-6.
  The manifestations of HHV-7 are similar to HHV-6 infection.

- *HHV-8*: HHV-8 is associated with mucocutaneous Kaposi's sarcoma and has also been linked with sarcoidosis.

Orofacial involvement is most commonly encountered in infections caused by herpes simplex and herpes zoster.[4, 5] Herpes infections are usually recognised on the basis of clinical signs and symptoms. Definitive diagnosis requires appropriate investigations including serological tests to detect viral antigens and host antibodies.[3] Most herpes infections in otherwise healthy patients are self-limiting and can be managed with conservative measures aimed at achieving symptomatic relief, as described in Section 8.2. However, herpes infections in patients with additional risk factors such as old age, immunosuppression due to an underlying medical condition or immunosuppressive medication require systemic antiviral therapy.[3, 4] Patients with these risk factors and/or those experiencing marked systemic involvement are best managed under specialist care in hospital settings, and dentists must refer these patients appropriately at the earliest.

8.2 TREATMENT PRINCIPLES OF HERPES VIRUS INFECTIONS

8.2.1 GENERAL MEASURES

- Improve personal and hand hygiene.

- Bed rest and isolation.

- Fluids to correct dehydration.

- Non-aspirin-based antipyretics and analgesics such as paracetamol to manage fever and pain.
  Use of aspirin-based analgesics in children and adolescents with viral infections can cause *Reye's syndrome* which can manifest with life-threatening complications such as cerebral oedema, seizures, liver damage and cardiorespiratory arrest. Therefore, aspirin-based analgesics should be avoided.

8.2.2 ANTIVIRAL THERAPY

- *Early treatment*: When indicated, initiate antiviral therapy at the earliest. Antiviral medications work best when they are started early in the course of the infection, ideally within the first 48 hours of symptoms.

- *Duration of treatment*: The duration of antiviral therapy depends on the severity of the infection and the individual's response to treatment. In most cases, treatment is continued until the symptoms have resolved.

- *Suppressive therapy*: For individuals who experience frequent or severe oral herpes outbreaks, daily antiviral therapy can be used to suppress the virus and reduce the frequency and severity of outbreaks.

- *Combination therapy*: In some cases, combination therapy with multiple antiviral medications may be used to improve the effectiveness of treatment and reduce risks of drug resistance.

Systemic antiviral therapy should be undertaken by dentists only if they are experienced in providing such treatment, otherwise it may be best to refer the patients to specialists in oral medicine and/or medical experts at a local hospital.

8.2.3 ORAL CARE

- Maintain good oral hygiene with soft toothbrush and antimicrobial mouthwashes.

- Soft, non-irritant diet.

- If oral ulcers are present, symptomatic relief may be achieved with topical analgesics and anaesthetics (see Chapter 12).

- Dental treatment may be postponed until the infection has subsided.

8.2.4 PREVENTION

- Avoid close contact with individuals who have active herpes lesions.

- Maintain optimal hygiene.

- Use barrier methods during sexual activity.

- *Vaccination*: Currently, there are no licensed vaccines for HSV 1, 2. Vaccines against herpes zoster are approved by FDA and include Zostavax (live-attenuated vaccine) and Shingrix (recombinant zoster vaccine).[5] These are indicated for people over 50 years.

8.3 ANTIVIRAL AGENTS FOR HERPES VIRUS INFECTIONS

Antiviral agents used to treat herpes infections include nucleoside analogues such as, acyclovir, famciclovir, valacyclovir and penciclovir.[1, 6] Other agents include antiviral peptides such as docosanol.[7]

Mechanism of action: Nucleoside analogues, such as acyclovir, valaciclovir and famciclovir, work by inhibiting viral DNA synthesis.[8] They are structurally similar to natural nucleosides, which are the building blocks of DNA. These drugs have a greater affinity for viral enzymes than for host enzymes. During viral replication, the nucleoside analogue is incorporated into the viral DNA instead of the natural nucleosides, which prevents viral DNA synthesis.

8.3.1 ACYCLOVIR

Acyclovir, a purine nucleoside analogue, is an effective antiviral drug used primarily against herpes viruses.[8] Acyclovir has low oral bioavailability (15–30%) and short half-life and needs to be administered every 3–4 hours.[9]

Indications: Herpes simplex and herpes zoster infection.

Side effects: Headaches, nausea, vomiting, diarrhoea, photosensitivity.

Cautions: Side effects may be more marked in people over 65 years.

COMMERCIAL PREPARATIONS:

Zovirax®

   Tablets/Capsules, acyclovir 200 mg, 400 mg, 800 mg
   Suspension, acyclovir 200 mg/5 mL, 400 mg/mL
   Intravenous infusion, powder for reconstitution acyclovir (as sodium salt) 250 mg, 500 mg
   Cream, acyclovir 5%

ROUTE OF ADMINISTRATION AND DOSE:

Oral

   Herpes simplex
      Treatment: 200 mg (400 mg in immunocompromised or if absorption impaired) 5 times daily, usually for 5–7 days. Child 15 mg/kg.
      Prevention of recurrence: 200 mg 4 times daily or 400 mg twice daily; child 15 mg/kg.
      Prophylaxis in immunocompromised: 200–400 mg 4 times daily; child 15 mg/kg.

   Varicella zoster
      Treatment: 800 mg 5 times daily for 7 days; child 20 mg/kg.
      iv Infusion.
      Intravenous administration should be restricted to specialist settings only.

Topical

   Acyclovir cream (5%) is indicated for the treatment of initial and recurrent labial and genital herpes simplex infections.
   Administration: Apply to lesions every 4 hours (5 times daily), started at first sign of attack.
   Side effects: Transient stinging or burning; occasionally erythema or drying of the skin.
   Cautions: Avoid contact with eyes and mucous membranes

8.3.2 VALACICLOVIR

Valaciclovir: It is a prodrug of acyclovir that is converted in the body to acyclovir and has better oral bioavailability (54%) and longer half-life than acyclovir.[9]

Indications: Treatment of herpes simplex and herpes zoster infections of skin and mucous membranes including initial and recurrent genital herpes.

Side effects: Similar to acyclovir.

Cautions: Renal impairment; pregnancy and breastfeeding; maintain adequate hydration.

COMMERCIAL PREPARATIONS:
Valtrex®
   Tablets, valaciclovir (as hydrochloride) 500 mg

ROUTE OF ADMINISTRATION AND DOSE:
Oral
 Herpes simplex: First episode 500 mg twice daily for 5 days (up to 10 days if severe); recurrent infection 500 mg twice daily for 5 days. Child 20 mg/kg.
 Herpes zoster: 1 g 3 times daily for 7 days.

8.3.3 PENCICLOVIR

Penciclovir is guanine nucleoside analogue acyclovir and is similar to acyclovir in its antiviral activity and pharmacological effects. Despite the low potency of penciclovir (100-fold less than acyclovir) in inhibiting DNA polymerase, it has a longer intracellular half-life (7–20 hours) than acyclovir.[7]

Indications: Treatment of labial herpes simplex infection.

Side effects: Transient stinging, burning, numbness.

Cautions: Avoid contact with eyes and mucous membranes.

COMMERCIAL PREPARATIONS:

Denavir®/Vectavir®
 Cream, penciclovir 1%.

ROUTE OF ADMINISTRATION AND DOSE:

Apply penciclovir cream (1%) to lesions of herpes labialis every 2 hours during waking hours for 4 days, starting at the first sign of the attack.

8.3.4 FAMCICLOVIR

Famciclovir is a prodrug of guanine nucleoside analogue *penciclovir*, which is converted to penciclovir in the body after oral use. In addition to its antiherpetic effects, Famciclovir also has activity against hepatitis-B virus.[6]

Indications: Treatment of herpes zoster, acute genital herpes simplex and suppression of recurrent genital herpes.

Side effects: Nausea, vomiting, headache; dizziness, confusion, rashes.

Cautions: Renal impairment; pregnancy and breastfeeding.

COMMERCIAL PREPARATIONS:

Famvir®
 Tablets, famciclovir 125 mg, 250 mg, 500 mg

ROUTE OF ADMINISTRATION AND DOSE:

Oral
 Recurrent herpes labialis: Adults – 1500 mg as a single dose.
 Shingles: 500 mg every 8 hours for 7 days.
 Recurrent herpes infections in HIV-infected adults—500 mg twice daily for 7 days.

8.3.5 DOCOSANOL

Docosanol (also known as behenyl alcohol) is a saturated fatty alcohol, which inhibits a broad range of lipid-enveloped viruses including HSV-1 and HSV-2. Docosanol is approved by the FDA as an over-the-counter antiviral agent for the management of herpes labialis.[7]

Mechanism of action: Docosanol inhibits and prevents herpes virus replication through inhibiting viral envelop fusion with the human host cell.[7]

Indications: Herpes labialis.

Side effects: Well tolerated. Potential side effects may include skin irritation and stinging.

Cautions: Pregnancy and breastfeeding.

COMMERCIAL PREPARATIONS:

Abreva®

Cream, doconazole 10%.

ROUTE OF ADMINISTRATION AND DOSE:

Apply doconazole cream (10%) to lesions of herpes labialis every 4–5 times daily, starting at the first sign of attack.

8.4 MISCELLANEOUS VIRAL INFECTIONS

8.4.1 HUMAN PAPILLOMA VIRUS

Human papilloma virus (HPV) is a double-stranded DNA virus and is the most common sexually transmitted viral infection. Over 200 types of HPV have been identified. Apart from genital warts, HPV infection can result in oral warts which present as cauliflower-like spiked lesions on the oral mucosa. Warts can be treated with surgery, laser or cryotherapy. Medical options include topical treatment with imiquimod, podofilox and 5-fluorouracil. General dental practice settings are not suitable for medical or surgical management of warts, and patients should be referred to specialists.

HPV is also associated with cervical and oropharyngeal carcinomas. HPV-16 is considered the most common type of HPV associated with oropharyngeal carcinoma. Suspicious oral lesions should be referred to an oral and maxillofacial surgeon for a second opinion. Prevention of HPV-associated carcinomas can be achieved with HPV vaccination, ideally prior to exposure to the virus, usually at the age of 11–12 years.[1, 2] Although the HPV vaccine is highly effective, it does not protect against all HPV types. Therefore, practicing safe sexual behaviours and undergoing routine screenings remain important components of overall HPV prevention.

8.4.2 HAND, FOOT AND MOUTH DISEASE

Hand, foot and mouth disease (HFMD) is caused by several different types of viruses from the Enterovirus genus, most commonly Enterovirus 71 (EV71) and Coxsackievirus A16 (CA16).[2] The infection commonly affects the children and presents with fever, sore throat and skin rashes on the hands, feet and mouth and may also involve the buttocks and genitals. The condition is usually self-limiting and managed with improvement in personal hygiene, frequent hand washing, limiting contact and non-aspirin-based antipyretics and analgesics such as paracetamol.[2, 3]

8.4.3 HERPANGINA

Herpangina is a viral illness caused by several types of viruses from the Enterovirus genus, most commonly Coxsackievirus A.[1] It typically affects children and is characterised by small, vesicles which rupture to leave painful ulcers on the posterior palate, tongue and pharynx. Systemic symptoms include fever, headache, sore throat and difficulty in swallowing. The condition is usually self-limiting and managed with non-aspirin-based antipyretics and analgesics such as paracetamol, topical anaesthetics/analgesics and non-irritant food.

8.4.4 MUMPS

Mumps is an acute viral infection caused by a paramyxovirus, a member of the Rubulavirus family.[10] The condition is spread through respiratory droplets and typically affects young children. It presents with fever, headache, muscle aches, fatigue and parotitis. Mumps leads to a painful swelling of the parotid glands (parotitis) initially unilaterally. Eventually bilateral parotid involvement is seen in most cases. The condition may be associated with varying degrees of xerostomia. One of the recognised complications is orchitis (testicular inflammation) which can cause male infertility. Patients experiencing testicular pain or swelling should be referred to medical colleagues for further evaluation and management. Other complications include oophoritis (inflammation of the ovaries in females), pancreatitis, encephalitis and meningitis. The condition is usually self-limiting and managed with bed rest, fluids to correct dehydration, limiting contact, and non-aspirin-based antipyretics and analgesics such as paracetamol. Prevention of mumps is primarily through vaccination with the MMR (measles, mumps, rubella) vaccine.[10]

RESOURCES

RESOURCES FOR DENTAL PROFESSIONALS

AAOM (The American Association of Oral Medicine). Dental care for the patient with an oral herpetic lesion. https://www.aaom.com/index.php?option=com_content&view=article&id=161:clinical-practice-statement--dental-care-for-the-patient-with-an-oral-herpetic-lesion&catid=24:clinical-practice-statement (accessed 25 February 2024).

RESOURCES FOR DENTAL PATIENTS

Mayo Clinic. Cold sore. https://www.mayoclinic.org/diseases-conditions/cold-sore/symptoms-causes/syc-20371017 (accessed 25 February 2024).

John Hopkins Medicine. Oral herpes. https://www.hopkinsmedicine.org/health/conditions-and-diseases/herpes-hsv1-and-hsv2/oral-herpes#:~:text=The%20best%20treatment%20for%20oral,%2Dcounter%20anti%2Dinflammatory%20agents (accessed 25 February 2024).

REFERENCES

1. McCullough, M.J. and Savage, N.W. (2005). Oral viral infections and the therapeutic use of antiviral agents in dentistry. *Australian Dental Journal* 50: S31–S35.

2. Bandara, H.M.H.N. and Samaranayake, L.P. (2019). Viral, bacterial, and fungal infections of the oral mucosa: types, incidence, predisposing factors, diagnostic algorithms, and management. *Periodontology 2000* 80: 148–176.

3. Clarkson, E., Mashkoor, F., and Abdulateef, S. (2017). Oral viral infections: diagnosis and management. *Dental Clinics of North America* 61: 353–363.

4. Ballyram, R., Wood, N.H., Khammissa, R.A.G. et al. (2016). Oral diseases associated with human herpes viruses: aetiology, clinical features, diagnosis and management: clinical review. *South African Dental Journal* 71 (6): 253–259.

5. Harbecke, R., Cohen, J.I., and Oxman, M.N. (2021). Herpes zoster vaccines. *The Journal of Infectious Diseases* 224 (Suppl. 4): S429–S442.

6. Poole, C.L. and James, S.H. (2018). Antiviral therapies for herpesviruses: current agents and new directions. *Clinical Therapeutics* 40: 1282–1298.

7. Hammer, K.D.P., Dietz, J., Shien Lo, T., and Johnson, E.M. (2018). A systematic review on the efficacy of topical acyclovir, penciclovir, and docosanol for the treatment of herpes simplex labialis. *EMJ Dermatology* 6: 118–123.

8. Kłysik, K., Pietraszek, A., Karewicz, A., and Nowakowska, M. (2018). Acyclovir in the treatment of herpes viruses – a review. *Current Medicinal Chemistry* 27 (24): 4118–4137.

9. Abdalla, S., Briand, C., Oualha, M. et al. (2020). Population pharmacokinetics of intravenous and oral acyclovir and oral valacyclovir in pediatric population to optimize dosing regimens. *Antimicrobial Agents and Chemotherapy* 64 (12): e01426-20.

10. Bin, S.S., Chang, H.L., and Chen, K.T. (2020). Current status of mumps virus infection: epidemiology, pathogenesis, and vaccine. *International Journal of Environmental Research and Public Health* 17: 1686.

CHAPTER 9 Antifungal Agents

Sadeq Ali Al-Maweri and Kamran Ali

Qatar University, QU Health, College of Dental Medicine, Doha, Qatar

9.1 INTRODUCTION

Fungal infections of orofacial soft tissues are well recognised and may be associated with significant discomfort and morbidity. There has been a global increase in the incidence of oral fungal infections, and this may be related to more widespread use of immunosuppressive medications. Although a variety of fungal infections can involve the oral cavity, infections caused by *Candida* spp. are the most common[1]. Infections by *Candida* spp. are opportunistic infections, most commonly caused by *candida albicans*, though other *Candida* spp. are also implicated. Although candidiasis may be observed in healthy individuals, immunosuppression, anaemia, antibiotic use, smoking, and poor oral hygiene, denture wearing and a diet rich in refined carbohydrates are recognised predisposing factors[2, 3]. Common local and systemic predisposing factors for oral candidiasis are summarised in Table 9.1.

There are many clinical types of oral candidiasis including acute pseudomembranous candidiasis (oral thrush), acute atrophic candidiasis (antibiotic sore mouth), chronic atrophic candidiasis (denture stomatitis), angular cheilitis, central papillary atrophy (median rhomboid glossitis), hyperplastic candidiasis and chronic mucocutaneous forms. The management of oral candidiasis includes addressing the underlying systemic/local predisposing factors and use of antifungal medications[4].

9.2 TREATMENT PRINCIPLES OF ORAL CANDIDIASIS

- *General measures*
  - Correction/control of underlying systemic predisposing factors such as anaemia, diabetes mellitus and immunosuppression.
  - Address local predisposing factors (high dietary content of refined sugars, smoking and xerostomia).
  - Improve physical and oral hygiene including denture hygiene.
  - Avoid injudicious use of antibiotics and prescribe only when absolutely necessary (see Chapters 4 and 7).
  - Patients using corticosteroid inhalers for chronic conditions such as asthma should be advised to brush and rinse their mouth with water following each application of an inhaler. Also, seek advice from the patient's physician regarding a non-steroidal inhaler, or consider use of a spacer device.

- *Antifungal therapy*
  - *Early treatment*: Early treatment is preferable for better treatment outcomes.
  - *Duration of treatment*: The duration of antifungal therapy depends on the severity of the infection and the individual's response to treatment. In most cases, treatment is continued at least 48 hours after the resolution of signs and symptoms.
  - *Route of treatment*: For mild–moderate cases, topical antifungals are recommended.

Clinical Dental Pharmacology, First Edition. Edited by Kamran Ali.
© 2024 John Wiley & Sons Ltd. Published 2024 by John Wiley & Sons Ltd.

Table 9.1 Predisposing Factors for Oral Candidiasis

Local factors	Systemic factors
• Poor oral hygiene • Xerostomia • Smoking • Diet rich in refined carbohydrates • Dentures	• Extremes of age • Anaemia • Poorly controlled diabetes mellitus • HIV infection • Immunosuppressive medications such as steroids, cyclosporine and azathioprine. • Broad-spectrum antibiotic therapy • Cancer • Chemotherapy • Radiation therapy for head and neck cancer • Major surgery

- Systemic antifungal therapy is indicated for severe cases, non-responsive to topical therapy and in immunosuppressed patients. It is important to consult with the patient's physician to monitor hepatic and renal function tests when using systemic azole antifungals.
- Combination topical therapy may be effective in chronic oral candidiasis.
- Patients with non-resolving lesions should be referred to a specialist in oral medicine and/or an appropriate medical expert at a local hospital. This is particularly important if there is a suspicion regarding the diagnosis and possibility of suspicious lesions associated with premalignant/malignant changes. Also, burning mouth syndrome may present with oral candidiasis.

***ORAL CARE*:**

- Maintain good oral hygiene with soft toothbrush and antimicrobial mouthwashes such as chlorhexidine gluconate 0.12%.

- Provide dietary advice to limit the amount and frequency of refined carbohydrates.

- If lesions are associated with pain or discomfort, symptomatic relief may be achieved with topical analgesics and anaesthetics.

- Consider providing smoking cessation advice to patients who smoke.

- Manage dry mouth (see Chapter 13).

- Denture care in patients with denture stomatitis (DS).
  - Meticulous oral hygiene including prosthesis care is important to achieve resolution of DS.
  - Brush the hard palate for 2 minutes, 3 times a day, with soft toothbrush bristles and water.
    - During the day, brush the dentures for 2 minutes, 3 times a day, with a denture brush and neutral, non-abrasive liquid soap.
    - Before going to bed at night, soak the dentures in 150 mL of 0.25–0.5% sodium hypochlorite for 10–20 minutes (acrylic dentures only) followed by overnight storage of dentures in fresh, clean water at room temperature and leave the denture out during night. Alternatively, dentures may be rinsed in chlorhexidine 0.12% mouthwash.
    - Apply topical antifungal medication on the palate and denture (see the following section on Miconazole).
    - Evaluate the dentures and adjust/replace as required.

- *Angular cheilitis*:
  - Often caused by a combination of *Candida* spp. and *Streptococcus* spp./*Staphylococcus* spp. Therefore, the treatment may benefit from drugs with additional antibacterial activity, such as miconazole (see the following section on Miconazole).

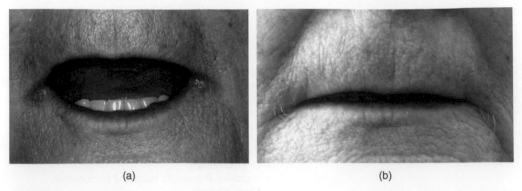

(a)　　　　　　　　　　　　　　　(b)

FIGURE 9.1 An elderly lady with bilateral angular cheilitis (a). Complete resolution achieved with oral fluconazole for 10 days (b)

- Patients should avoid licking the lesion to minimise the risk of superinfection with salivary bacteria.
- Non-responsive cases may benefit from a combination of miconazole and hydrocortisone or oral antifungals such as fluconazole (Figure 9.1).
- If angular cheilitis is observed in patients with dentures, evaluate the dentures and adjust/replace as required.

9.3 COMMON ANTIFUNGAL AGENTS

Antifungals are often used for the treatment of oral candidiasis and other fungal infections. Common antifungals include the following classes of drugs:

- *Polyenes*: Nystatin and amphotericin B.

- *Azoles*

  Triazoles: Fluconazole and itraconazole.
  Imidazoles: Clotrimazole, miconazole, ketoconazole and tioconazole.

9.3.1 POLYENE ANTIFUNGAL AGENTS

Mechanism of action: Target to sterols in the fugal cell membranes, specifically the ergosterol component present in fungal cell membranes but absent in mammalian cells. This disrupts the fungal cell membrane, leading to loss of cellular macromolecules and ions, producing irreversible damage.

Nystatin

Nystatin, a polyene antifungal, is an effective antifungal drug used primarily against oral candidiasis.

Indications: Oropharyngeal and perioral candidiasis in immunocompetent as well as immunocompromised patients.

Side effects: Generally well-tolerated; mild gastrointestinal disturbances (nausea, vomiting and diarrhoea). Local side effects include bitter taste.

COMMERCIAL PREPARATIONS:

Mycostatin®

Suspension, nystatin 100,000 U/mL
Powder, nystatin 100,000
Lozenges: Nystatin 200,000 U
Ointment: Nystatin 100,000 U/g

ROUTE OF ADMINISTRATION AND DOSE:

2–3 mL of a 100,000 U/mL (teaspoon) of nystatin suspension is placed in the mouth, swished and held for 3–5 minutes before swallowing, 4 times daily for around 10 days or at least 48 hours after resolution of the lesions.

Or

One or two 200,000 U/mL lozenges can be used every 6 hours for 10 days or at least 48 hours after remission of the lesion.

Nystatin cream applied 4 times/day in angular cheilitis.

Prophylaxis in susceptible patients: 2–3 mL of a 100,000 U/mL of nystatin suspension is placed in the mouth, swished and held for 3–5 minutes before swallowing, 4 times daily for around 10 days or at least 48 hours after remission of the lesion.

Amphotericin B

Amphotericin B, a polyene antibiotic, is an effective antifungal drug against a broad spectrum of fungal infections including Candidiasis. Amphotericin B is not absorbed from mucocutaneous tissues, and thus it is administered systemically via intravenous infusion.

Given its toxicity and other side effects, amphotericin B has limited clinical use in general dental practice settings and is reserved for the treatment refractory/life-threatening cases in specialist settings.

Indications: Severe oropharyngeal candidiasis cases not responsive to other systemic antifungal medications.

Side effects: *Allergy,* fever, hypotension, delirium, abdominal pain, anorexia, nausea, vomiting, headache, nephrotoxicity, thrombophlebitis, and also hypochromic, normocytic anaemia.

Cautions: High toxicity; hepatic and renal function tests and monitoring of blood counts is required.

COMMERCIAL PREPARATIONS:

Fungilin®

Lozenges, amphotericin B 10 mg
Oral Suspension, amphotericin B 100 mg/mL

ROUTE OF ADMINISTRATION AND DOSE:

Dissolve 1 lozenge slowly in the mouth 4 times/day (10–14 days).

Oral suspension, administer 1 mL through a pipette after food and retain near lesions 4 times/day (up to 14 days). Continue for at least 48 hours after resolution of lesions.

9.3.2 AZOLE ANTIFUNGAL AGENTS

Mechanism of action: Azole antifungals work by inhibiting the synthesis of ergosterol, a vital component of the fungal cell membrane. This involves targeting an enzyme, lanosterol 14 α-demethylase, which is responsible for converting lanosterol into ergosterol in fungal cells. As a result, the integrity of cell membrane is impaired leading to disruption of vital processes in fungal cells.

Cautions: Azole antifungals interact with warfarin and statins, potentiating their effects. Therefore, azole antifungals discussed in the following text and should be avoided in patients taking these medications.

Topical Azole Antifungals

Miconazole   Miconazole is a synthetic imidazole antifungal drug, used primarily for the treatment of infection by *Candida* spp. It is also effective against gram-positive cocci and is therefore indicated in the management of angular cheilitis.

Indications: Treatment of angular cheilitis and DS.

Side effects: Nausea, vomiting, diarrhoea, chills, alteration in taste, dry mouth.

Cautions: Avoid during pregnancy; do not prescribe to patients taking warfarin or statins; do not use in children under 2 years of age.

COMMERCIAL PREPARATIONS:

Daktarin®

Oromucosal gel, miconazole 20 mg/mL

ROUTE OF ADMINISTRATION AND DOSE:

Apply a small pea-sized amount (2.5 mL) over the affected area 4 times/day after food. The treatment should be continued for 7 days after complete remission of the lesions.

Denture stomatitis: Applied to the fitting surface of an upper denture before placing the denture in the mouth.

COMPOUND PREPARATIONS:

Daktacort®

2/1% w/w cream, miconazole nitrate (2%) with hydrocortisone (1%) cream
Daktacort 2/1% w/w ointment, miconazole nitrate (2%) with hydrocortisone (1%) cream

Useful for the treatment of refractory angular cheilitis. Apply to the angles of mouth twice daily for up to 7 days. Creams are best used on wet surfaces, while ointments are suitable for use on dry surfaces.

Clotrimazole   Clotrimazole is a synthetic imidazole antifungal drug, used primarily for the management of mucocutaneous candidiasis. It is used topically only.

Indications: Treatment of all forms of mild to moderate oral candidiasis.

Side effects: Nausea, vomiting, gastric upset; and mucosal irritation and inching.

Cautions: Avoid during pregnancy.

COMMERCIAL PREPARATIONS:

Mycelex®

Troches/lozenges, clotrimazole 10 mg

Mycelex

Cream, clotrimazole 1%

Mycelex

Solution, clotrimazole 1%

ROUTE OF ADMINISTRATION AND DOSE:

10 mg troche dissolved in the mouth 4–5 times daily for 10–14 days.

Mycelex cream 1% to be applied 3–4 times daily for 10–14 days.

Ketoconazole Ketoconazole is a synthetic azole antifungal medication. It is the first systemic azole medication approved for deep systemic mycoses. However, it has high toxicity and frequent drug interactions.

Indications: Topical ketoconazole can be used for cutaneous candidiasis. However, it should not be applied in the mouth.

Side effects: Headache, dizziness, mood changes, nausea, vomiting and gastric upset, hepatotoxicity.

Cautions: Should be used with caution in patients with insufficient hepatic function, history of cardiac diseases and during pregnancy.

COMMERCIAL PREPARATIONS:

Nizoral®

2% cream

ROUTE OF ADMINISTRATION AND DOSE:

Clean and thoroughly dry the affected area on the skin and apply Nizoral 2% cream once or twice daily. The duration of therapy varies depending on response to therapy but may require 2–6 weeks for the infection to resolve.

Oral Azole Antifungals

Fluconazole Fluconazole is a synthetic triazole antifungal drug, used primarily for the treatment of infections with *Candida* spp. (and other fungi) which are resistant to topical therapy. It is also suitable for the treatment of fungal infections in immunocompromised patients.

Indications: Oropharyngeal candidiasis (including invasive form); prevention of candidiasis in immunocompromised.

Side effects: Nausea, vomiting, gastric pain, headache and rashes. Rarely allergy and hypersensitivity reactions.

Cautions: Avoid during pregnancy; do not prescribe to patients taking warfarin or statins.

COMMERCIAL PREPARATIONS:

Diflucan®

Tablets 50 mg, 100 mg, 150 mg, 200 mg
Diflucan oral suspension for reconstitution with water, 10; 40 mg/mL

ROUTE OF ADMINISTRATION AND DOSE:

50 mg orally daily (100 in more resistant cases) for 7–14 days in oropharyngeal candidiasis; for 14 days in oral atrophic candidiasis associated with DS.

Child: 6 months–11 years 3–6 mg/kg on first day and then 3 mg/kg (max. 50 mg) daily; 12–17 years 50 mg daily.

Itraconazole Itraconazole is a water-insoluble, broad-spectrum triazole antifungal.

Indications: Oropharyngeal candidiasis.

Side effects: Headache, mild gastrointestinal disturbances, raised liver enzymes, peripheral neuropathy (therapy should be discontinued), rare rash, hypersensitivity and allergic reactions. Hair loss after prolonged use is also reported.

Cautions: Hepatorenal impairment; raised liver enzymes.

COMMERCIAL PREPARATIONS:

Sporanox®

100 mg capsules
Sporanox oral liquid 10 mg/mL

ROUTE OF ADMINISTRATION AND DOSE:

Capsules: 100–200 mg capsule once daily for 2 weeks.

Liquid/solution: 10 mL to be swished for 2–3 minutes and then swallowed twice/day; do not rinse afterwards.

Ketoconazole Oral ketoconazole is reserved for refractory oropharyngeal candidiasis and due to its high toxicity, it is best prescribed in specialist settings.

9.4 OTHER ORAL FUNGAL INFECTIONS

9.4.1 HISTOPLASMOSIS

Histoplasmosis is a rare deep fungal infection of the lung caused by *Histoplasma capsulatum*. Oral manifestations of histoplasmosis are relatively rare and can present as solitary long-standing ulcerative or erosive lesion on the tongue palate or buccal/labial mucosae. The lesions mimic malignant ulcers. Management of histoplasmosis is best done in specialist settings and involves the use of systemic itraconazole along with amphotericin B.

9.4.2 BLASTOMYCOSIS

Blastomycosis is an endemic fungal infection caused by Blastomyces dermatitidis. It is a deep infection which mainly involves the lungs, cutaneous, as well as nervous, and genitourinary tissues. Oral involvement in disseminated blastomycosis include indurated ulcerative lesions mimicking oral squamous cell carcinoma. Acute and mild cases of blastomycosis are mostly self-limiting. Moderate to severe cases require systemic antifungal therapy under specialist care.

RESOURCES

RESOURCES FOR DENTAL PROFESSIONALS

Scottish Dental Clinical Effectiveness Programme (SDCP). Drug prescribing for dentistry. https://www.sdcep.org.uk/published-guidance/drug-prescribing/ (accessed 25 February 2024).

Ng, S. (2013). Managing patients with oral candidiasis. *Journal of the Canadian Dental Association* 79: d122. https://jcda.ca/article/d122 (accessed 25 February 2024).

RESOURCES FOR DENTAL PATIENTS

Cleveland Clinic. Candidiasis. https://my.clevelandclinic.org/health/diseases/23198-candidiasis (accessed 25 February 2024).

Mayo Clinic. Oral thrush. https://www.mayoclinic.org/diseases-conditions/oral-thrush/symptoms-causes/syc-20353533 (accessed 25 February 2024).

REFERENCES

1. Bandara, H.M.H.N. and Samaranayake, L.P. (2019). Viral, bacterial, and fungal infections of the oral mucosa: types, incidence, predisposing factors, diagnostic algorithms, and management. *Periodontology 2000* 80: 148–176.

2. Al-Maweri, S., Al-Sufyani, G., Tarakji, B. et al. (2015). Oral mucosal lesions in elderly dental patients in Sana'a, Yemen. *Journal of International Society of Preventive & Community Dentistry* 5 (7): S12.

3. Hato, H., Sakata, K.I., Sato, J. et al. (2022). Factor associated with oral candidiasis caused by co-infection of *Candida albicans* and *Candida glabrata*: a retrospective study. *Journal of Dental Sciences* 17 (3): 1458–1461.

4. Abuhajar, E., Ali, K., Zulfiqar, G. et al. (2023). Management of chronic atrophic candidiasis (denture stomatitis)—a narrative review. *International Journal of Environmental Research and Public Health* 20: 3029.

Miscellaneous Agents

Miscellaneous
Agents

SECTION

Oral Hygiene Agents: Toothpastes

CHAPTER 10

Manal Matoug-Elwerfelli[1] and Gail V.A. Douglas[2]

[1] *Qatar University, QU Health, College of Dental Medicine, Doha, Qatar*
[2] *School of Dentistry, University of Leeds, Leeds, UK*

10.1 INTRODUCTION

This chapter focusses on over-the-counter and prescription toothpastes (dentifrices) in the light of contemporary clinical guidelines and recommendations. Toothpastes used with a toothbrush remain the most widely used method of maintenance of oral hygiene globally. Based on the constituents, toothpastes are broadly classified into:

1. *Over-the-counter toothpastes*

   The main function of a toothpaste is to clean the teeth which falls under a cosmetic benefit. Claims such as 'cavity protection', 'cleans', 'protects', 'freshens breath', 'fights bacteria', 'fights tartar' and 'fights tooth decay' all of which are well-accepted and commonly used cosmetic claims.

   According to the UK and European Community law, the maximum fluoride concentration permitted in over-the-counter toothpastes is 0.15%, which is equivalent to 1500 ppm fluoride (ppm F)[1, 2]. FDI World Dental Federation also recommends that over-the-counter toothpastes with a fluoride concentration of between 1000 and 1500 ppm F[3].

2. *Prescription toothpastes*

   Toothpastes are classed as a medicine, available on a prescription, when their use is for the purpose of treating or preventing a specific dental disease. Specific indications include prevention/reduction of dental caries, management of dentine hypersensitivity and reduction in gingival bleeding. Such products generally require approval by a relevant regulator in the country such as Medicines and Healthcare Products Regulatory Agency (MHRA) in the United Kingdom and Food and Drug Administration in the United States prior to consumer availability.

   Toothpastes containing a fluoride concentration of greater than 1500 ppm F, such as 2800 and 5000 ppm F, are automatically classed as medicines and available on prescription only[1, 2].

10.2 COMPOSITION OF TOOTHPASTES

Toothpastes generally contain an abrasive or mixture thereof suspended in an aqueous humectant phase by means of a hydrocolloid. For a detailed review of toothpaste ingredients, the readers may consult a review by Lippert[4].

Clinical Dental Pharmacology, First Edition. Edited by Kamran Ali.
© 2024 John Wiley & Sons Ltd. Published 2024 by John Wiley & Sons Ltd.

- *Abrasives*: Help in the mechanical removal of plaque and stains from teeth. Common abrasives include calcium carbonate, silica and hydrated aluminium oxides.

- *Humectants*: Retain moisture and prevent toothpaste from drying out. Glycerine and sorbitol are commonly used humectants in toothpaste.

- *Binders and thickeners*: These ingredients give toothpaste its consistency and texture. They help in maintaining the proper form of toothpaste. Common binders and thickeners include cellulose gum, carrageenan and xanthan gum.

- *Detergents (surfactants)*: Create foam and help in the even distribution of toothpaste while brushing. Sodium lauryl sulphate (SLS) is a commonly used detergent. However, due to mucosal irritation with SLS, toothpastes free from SLS are gaining popularity and may be preferred for patients with sensitivity to SLS or those with xerostomia. Other examples of detergents include polyethylene glycol ethers of stearic acid and anionic alkyl sulfonates.

- *Flavouring agents*: These ingredients add flavour to toothpaste and help improve the taste. Common flavouring agents include spearmint, peppermint or other artificial flavours.

- *Sweeteners*: Enhance taste. Saccharin and sorbitol are commonly used sweeteners in toothpaste.

- *Preservatives*: Help maintain the stability and prevent microbial growth in toothpaste. Sodium benzoate and potassium sorbate are commonly used preservatives.

Mucosal irritation and contact allergy result from flavouring agents, detergents or other active ingredients in a toothpaste.

Additionally, toothpastes may also contain other active ingredients including one or more of the following:

- *Anticaries agents*:

   Fluorides: Help strengthen tooth enamel, inhibit the demineralisation of teeth and promote remineralisation. Commonly used agents include sodium fluoride, sodium monofluorophosphate and stannous fluoride.

- *Antiplaque/Antigingivitis agents*:

   Triclosan: It has antibacterial properties which help reduce plaque formation and gingivitis. Although Triclosan is approved by the FDA, it has been linked to disruption of thyroid gland function and antibiotic resistance. Hence, Triclosan-containing toothpastes are not available in the United States since 2019.

   Chlorhexidine: Antimicrobial agent which may be included in prescription strength toothpaste to treat severe gingivitis. It may be associated with risks of allergy and tooth discolouration with long-term use.

   Zinc citrate: Inhibits plaque formation and helps reduce gum inflammation.

- *Anticalculus agents*:

   Pyrophosphates: Bind to calcium phosphate crystals preventing phosphate ions from adsorption onto the crystal and inhibit calculus formation by preventing the mineralisation of plaque.

   Zinc citrate: Help to reduce calculus build-up by interfering with the calcification of plaque.

- *Antimalodour agents*:

   Zinc compounds: Zinc ions help neutralise volatile sulphur compounds responsible for bad breath.

   Chlorine dioxide: It has deodorising properties and helps reduce oral malodour.

10.3 FLUORIDATED TOOTHPASTES

Toothpastes containing a range of fluoride compounds with varying concentrations are currently available globally. Despite there being several types to date, insufficient evidence is available to recommend a specific fluoride formulation. Nevertheless, the concentration of fluoride is considered to be more relevant for clinical benefits[1, 2].

Tooth brushing with a fluoridated toothpaste is the most common delivery system for self-administration of fluoride and is effective in protection of the dental hard tissues against dental caries. According to the World Health Organization (WHO) guidelines, fluoridated toothpastes containing between 1000 and 1500 ppm F are recommended as a standard public oral health measure for the prevention of dental caries[5]. Toothpastes containing higher fluoride concentration are recommended for individuals at a high risk of dental caries such as those suffering from chronic xerostomia.

Dental fluorosis (dental enamel mineralisation defects) is a recognised dose-dependent side effect due to chronic ingestion of excessive amounts of fluoride (usually in the form of a toothpaste) during tooth formation in children.

Clinically, the recommendation of a specific fluoride concentration for an individual will largely depend on a caries risk assessment, as summarised in Tables 10.1 and 10.2 based on recognised professional guidelines[2, 6–8].

10.3.1 COMMERCIAL PRODUCTS

A plethora of toothpaste products containing standard fluoride concentrations for various age groups are available over the counter.

Toothpastes with high-fluoride concentrations require a prescription and the two most commonly used concentrations are 2800 and 5000 ppm F.

Table 10.1 Recommendations on Fluoridated Toothpastes for Individuals at low Risk of Dental Caries

American dental association/ american academy of paediatric dentistry/ american academy of paediatrics	Delivering better oral health united kingdom	European academy of paediatric dentistry	Australian research centre for population oral health guidelines
First tooth – up to 3 years: Smear amount (grain of rice) toothpaste (0.1 g of toothpaste or 0.1 mg F).	*First tooth – up to 3 years*: Smear amount of toothpaste containing at least 1000 ppm F.	*First tooth – up to 2 years*: Smear amount (0.125 g) of toothpaste containing 1000 ppm F.	*First tooth – up to 17 months*: Teeth should be cleaned by an adult, but without toothpaste.
3–6 years-old: Pea-sized amount (0.25 g of toothpaste or 0.25 mg F).	*3–6-years-old*: Pea-sized amount of toothpaste containing at least 1000 ppm F.	*2–6 years*: Pea-sized amount (0.25 g) of toothpaste containing 1000 ppm F.	*18 months–5-years-old*: Small pea-sized amount of toothpaste containing 500–550 ppm F (0.5–0.55 mg/g F).
	From 7 years – up to 18 years: Brush teeth with toothpaste containing between 1350 and 1500 ppm F.	*Over 6 years*: Full length of brush (0.5–1.0 g) of toothpaste containing 1450 ppm F.	*6-years-old and older*: Fluoridated toothpaste containing 1000–1500 ppm F (1–1.5 mg/g F).
	Adults: Brush teeth with toothpaste containing between 1350 and 1500 ppm F.		

Table 10.2 Recommendations on Fluoridated Toothpastes for Individuals at High Risk of Dental Caries

American dental association/ american academy of paediatric dentistry/ american academy of paediatrics	Delivering better oral health united kingdom	European academy of paediatric dentistry	Australian research centre for population oral health guidelines[a]
Not specified	*First tooth – up to 3 years*: Apply a smear amount of toothpaste (0.1 mL) containing between 1350 and 1500 ppm F.	*First tooth – up to 2 years*: Not specified.	Children: Variable, as needed, based on advice by a dental professional or trained health professional.
	3–6-years-old: Apply a pea-sized amount of toothpaste (0.25 mL) containing between 1350 and 1500 ppm F.	*2–6 years*: Toothpaste containing more than 1000 + ppm F may be considered.	
	7 years to 18 years: Consider daily fluoride mouthrinse (0.05% NaF; 230ppm F) at a different time to brushing		
	Other options: 10 years and older: Prescription of toothpaste 2800 ppm F.	*Over 6 years*: Not specified.	*Teenagers and adults*: Prescription of toothpaste containing 5000 ppm F.
	Over 16 years: Prescription of toothpaste either 2800 or 5000 ppm F.		

As a consensus, all guidelines recommend supervised tooth brushing for children, brushing teeth twice a day and spit don't rinse.

[a] Either high-risk individuals or who do not consume fluoridated water[6].

- *Colgate Duraphat® Fluoride 2800 ppm Toothpaste*:

   1 g of toothpaste contains 2.8 mg fluoride, corresponding to 2800 ppm F, sodium fluoride, 0.619% w/w.
   Suitable for adults and children over 10 years with high risk of dental caries.
   Apply 1 cm using a toothbrush twice a day after meals.

- *Colgate Duraphat® Fluoride 5000 ppm Toothpaste*:

   1 g of toothpaste contains 5 mg fluoride (as sodium fluoride), corresponding to 5000 ppm F, sodium fluoride 1.1% w/w.
   Suitable for individuals 16 years and above with a high risk of dental caries.
   Apply 1 cm using a toothbrush twice a day after meals.

10.4 SPECIAL FORMULATION TOOTHPASTES

A variety of special toothpaste formulations have been developed to address specific dental conditions and needs. These include the following:

10.4.1 DESENSITISING TOOTHPASTES

Toothpastes containing an active desensitising agent are regarded as a convenient, cost-effective and non-invasive method to reduce pain related to dentine hypersensitivity. Most commonly, a

Table 10.3 Active Ingredients in Desensitising Toothpastes

Mechanism of action	Active ingredients
1. Disturbance of the neural response to stimulus	– Potassium salts such as potassium chloride and potassium nitrate are reported to decrease the excitability of the nerve, thus making the nerves unresponsive to a given stimulus (depolarisation).
2. Occlusion of dentinal tubules to block the flow of tubular fluid	– Fluoride compounds, such as sodium fluoride and stannous fluoride, form an insoluble precipitate (calcium fluoride), which creates a physical barrier and narrows the diameter of dentinal tubules thus reducing dentine permeability. – Oxalates such as potassium oxalate offers the advantage of dual mechanism, via nerve depolarisation and occluding dentinal tubules due to the deposition of calcium oxalate crystals. – Arginine (L-arginine) is a unique amino acid with an ability to reduce dentine permeability via occlusion of dental tubules.

twice daily application of toothpaste–containing specific formulations is recommended for the reduction/relief of dentine hypersensitivity[9]. The mechanism of action and active ingredients of desensitising toothpastes are summarised in Table 10.3.

10.4.2 WHITENING TOOTHPASTES

Toothpastes with reported claims of 'tooth whitening' are of high interest and demand by the public. Various ingredients have been added to over-the-counter and prescription-based toothpastes to aid the removal and/or prevent extrinsic stain formation. These include mechanical, chemical and optical agents, and a summary of the most commonly used whitening agents are presented in Table 10.4. However, the efficacy of whitening agents remains questionable. Additionally, there are safety concerns with some of the products in whitening toothpastes.

10.4.3 HERBAL TOOTHPASTES

Toothpastes based on natural products extracted from medicinal plants are popular amongst certain groups of consumers. The main bioactive crude extracts present in plant species include alkaloids, essential oils and polyphenols. The purported benefits of plant-based ingredients include reduced risk of side effects, as well as antibacterial, antioxidant, anti-inflammatory and anti-allergic properties.

Examples of common herbal ingredients added to toothpastes include:

- *Aloe vera* extract (Aloe genus)

- Cortex ilicis rotunda extract (a dehydrated bark of *Ilex rotunda* Thunb herb)

- *Eugenia uniflora* Linn extract (Surinam cherry)

- *Rosmarinus officinalis* Linn extract (rosemary)

- Green tea leaf extract (*Camellina sinensis* plant)

- Scutellaria baicalensis Georgi extract (Chinese skullcap root)

- *Azadirachta indica* extract (Neem plant)

- *Salvadora persica* (*Miswak tree*)

Table 10.4 Mode of Action of Whitening Toothpastes

Active agents	Examples
Mechanical agents	
Abrasives; rely on the physical removal of extrinsic stains	Alumina, calcium carbonate, calcium pyrophosphate, dicalcium phosphate dihydrate, hydrated silica, perlite, sodium bicarbonate, charcoal[a]
Chemical agents	
– Peroxides	– Hydrogen peroxide (oxidises intrinsic stain molecules and consequently changes their absorption spectra to become invisible to the naked eye). – Calcium peroxide – Sodium citrate
– Phosphates	– Sodium pyrophosphate – Sodium tripolyphosphate – Sodium hexametaphosphate (poly pyrophosphate)
– Enzymes	– Papain
– Optical agents	– Blue covarine (alters optical properties of the tooth with a shift from a yellow to blue colour tooth surface, gives a perception of tooth whiteness).

[a] Charcoal-based toothpastes are marketed as oral hygiene products, with added benefits such as 'tooth whitening[10, 11]. The lack of fluoride in many charcoal-based toothpastes is also a concern, as it may lead to an increased risk of dental caries. Moreover, tooth abrasion and sensitivity may be associated with regular/long-term use charcoal-based toothpastes. To date, there is insufficient scientific evidence to support the use of charcoal-based toothpastes.

However, further clinical evidence is required to support the routine use of herbal toothpastes.

10.4.4 MISCELLANEOUS FORMULATIONS

Modifications to standard toothpastes ingredients have also been made in attempts to meet specific patient expectations and concerns. Examples include:

- Mild or non-foaming (detergent-free) toothpastes
- Mild or non-flavouring toothpastes
- Fluoride-free toothpastes

10.5 SUMMARY

Given the available evidence, fluoride-based toothpastes are the mainstay of prevention of dental caries. Toothpastes with other active ingredients may be advised to patients depending on specific risks and clinical indication(s). Everyone must brush at least twice a day with a fluoridated toothpaste, last thing at night (usually just before bedtime) and at one other time in the day. Moreover, after brushing, rinsing with water should be avoided to maintain the topical effect of the fluoridated toothpaste. It is also imperative to reiterate the need for regular interdental cleaning using appropriate methods to reduce plaque accumulation on surface inaccessible to the standard toothbrush.

RESOURCES

RESOURCES FOR DENTAL PROFESSIONALS

Scottish Dental Clinical Effectiveness Program (2018). Prevention and management of dental caries in children, 2e. Section 7.2. www.sdcep.org.uk/media/2zbkrdkg/sdcep-prevention-and-management-of-dental-caries-in-children-2nd-edition.pdf (accessed February 2024).

Delivering Better Oral Health (2021). Chapter 13: Evidence base for recommendations in the summary guidance tables. https://www.gov.uk/government/publications/delivering-better-oral-health-an-evidence-based-toolkit-for-prevention (accessed February 2024).

RESOURCES FOR DENTAL PATIENTS

National Health Service. Healthy teeth and gums. https://www.nhs.uk/live-well/healthy-teeth-and-gums/how-to-keep-your-teeth-clean (accessed February 2024).

MouthHealthy. Toothpastes. American Dental Association. https://www.mouthhealthy.org/all-topics-a-z/toothpaste (accessed February 2024).

MouthHealthy. Fluoride. American Dental Association. https://www.mouthhealthy.org/all-topics-a-z/fluoride (accessed February 2024).

Cleveland Clinic. Oral hygiene. https://my.clevelandclinic.org/health/diseases/16914-oral-hygiene (accessed February 2024).

REFERENCES

1. SIGN138 (2014). Dental interventions to prevent caries in children—a national clinical guideline. www.sign.ac.uk/our-guidelines/dental-interventions-to-prevent-caries-in-children (accessed 5 May 2023).

2. Delivering Better Oral Health (2021). Chapter 13: Evidence base for recommendations in the summary guidance tables. https://www.gov.uk/government/publications/delivering-better-oral-health-an-evidence-based-toolkit-for-prevention/chapter-13-evidence-base-for-recommendations-in-the-summary-guidance-tables (accessed 5 May 2023).

3. FDI (2018). Promoting dental health through fluoride toothpaste. https://www.fdiworlddental.org/promoting-dental-health-through-fluoride-toothpaste (accessed 28 April 2023).

4. Lippert, F. (2013). An introduction to toothpaste - its purpose, history and ingredients. In: *Toothpastes. Monographs in Oral Science* (ed. C. van Loveren), 1–14. S. Karger AG.

5. World Health Organization (2019). *Preventing Disease through Healthy Environments: Inadequate or Excess Fluoride: A Major Public Health Concern*. Geneva: World Health Organization. WHO/CED/PHE/EPE/19.4.5.

6. Do, L. and Australian Research Centre for Population Oral Health (2020). Guidelines for use of fluorides in Australia: update 2019. *Australian Dental Journal* 65: 30–38.

7. American Dental Association (ADA) (2021). Toothpastes. https://www.ada.org/resources/research/science-and-research-institute/oral-health-topics/toothpastes (accessed 5 May 2023).

8. European Archives of Pediatric Dentistry: Guidelines on the use of fluoride for caries prevention in children: an updated EAPD policy document. https://link.springer.com/article/10.1007/s40368-019-00464-2 (accessed 19 February 2024).

9. Pollard, A.J., Khan, I., Davies, M. et al. (2023). Comparative efficacy of self-administered dentifrices for the management of dentine hypersensitivity - a systematic review and network meta-analysis. *Journal of Dentistry* 130: 104433.

10. Greenwall, L.H., Greenwall-Cohen, J., and Wilson, N.H. (2019). Charcoal-containing dentifrices. *British Dental Journal* 226: 697–700.

11. Brooks, J.K., Bashirelahi, N., and Reynolds, M.A. (2017). Charcoal and charcoal-based dentifrices: a literature review. *The Journal of the American Dental Association* 148: 661–670.

| CHAPTER 11 | # Oral Hygiene Agents: Mouthwashes |

Manal Matoug-Elwerfelli[1] and Gail V.A. Douglas[2]
[1] *Qatar University, QU Health, College of Dental Medicine, Doha, Qatar*
[2] *School of Dentistry, University of Leeds, Leeds, UK*

11.1 INTRODUCTION

Maintenance of oral hygiene with effective plaque control is critical to the prevention of common oral diseases such as dental caries and periodontal disease. To date, the most reliable method of plaque control is mechanical cleaning with a toothbrush and interdental cleaning aids such as dental floss and interdental brushes.

Mouthwashes (mouth rinses) are best used as adjuncts to maintain oral health and are mainly used in acute situations and during periods of interrupted hygiene (e.g., after periodontal surgery). Mouthwashes do not penetrate into the gingival crevice adequately, and they are primarily used for control of supragingival plaque. Fluoride-based mouthwashes are also helpful in the prevention of dental caries and can be used in high-risk patients. Finally, mouthwashes may be used for the management of oral hygiene in handicapped individuals, when adequate plaque control using mechanical measures effectively is compromised.

Although a wide variety of mouthwashes are available over-the-counter, use of prescription-only mouthwashes should be informed by specific clinical indications and an evaluation of the benefits and risks of a mouthwash. Considerations related to the prescription of mouthwashes are summarised as follows:

- Mouthwashes are adjuncts to oral hygiene and should not be used as a substitute to mechanical cleaning.

- Frequency of usage depends on the concentration of active ingredient (either daily, twice a day or weekly) as recommended by the manufacturer.

- After use, all mouthwashes should be spat out and never swallowed.

- Avoid eating, drinking, or rinse the mouth for at least 30 minutes after usage.

- Children using mouthwashes require adult supervision to avoid accidental swallowing and overdose.

- Patients using prescription mouthwashes for long periods need to be monitored for any side effects.

11.2 COMPOSITION OF MOUTHWASHES

Mouthwashes typically contain a variety of constituents, including detergents (surfactants), flavouring agents, colourants, preservatives and solvents such as water or alcohol. Water-based

---

Clinical Dental Pharmacology, First Edition. Edited by Kamran Ali.
© 2024 John Wiley & Sons Ltd. Published 2024 by John Wiley & Sons Ltd.

(alcohol-free) mouthwashes are preferred because alcohol can lead to dehydration of the oral mucosa leading to dryness which can aggravate the symptoms in patients with xerostomia (see Chapter 13). Alcohol can also lead to irritation and burning of the oral mucosa, especially in patients with mucosal inflammation and ulceration. Moreover, there is potential of alcohol abuse by individuals prone to alcohol addiction. Flavouring agents, detergents, preservatives or other ingredients in a mouthwash can also lead to mucosal irritation and contact allergy.

Active chemical agents in a mouthwash provide specific oral health benefits. The most common active agents in mouthwashes include the following:

- *Fluoride*:
  Fluoride is added to some mouthwashes to strengthen tooth enamel and help prevent dental caries.

- *Antiseptics/antimicrobials*:
  These agents help control microbial growth in the mouth, prevent or control oral infections, reduce inflammation and manage periodontal disease.
  - *Chlorhexidine gluconate*: An effective broad-spectrum antimicrobial agent for treating periodontal disease[1].
  - *Povidone-iodine*: Releases free iodine which has a broad-spectrum antimicrobial activity.
  - *Cetylpyridinium chloride (CPC)*: A cationic quaternary ammonium compound that binds to bacterial surfaces causing disruption to the cell membrane and metabolism. It is used to reduce bacteria and minimise halitosis.

- *Antiplaque/antigingivitis agents*:
  These agents help control plaque formation and reduce gum inflammation.
  - *Essential oils (e.g., thymol, eucalyptol, menthol and methyl salicylate)*: These oils have antimicrobial properties and are commonly used in mouthwashes to inhibit plaque growth and reduce gum inflammation.
  - *Astringents*: Astringents provide a tightening or drying effect on oral tissues.

- *Desensitising agents*:
  These agents help reduce dentine sensitivity and include potassium nitrate and various fluoride salts.

- *Oxygenating agents*:
  These agents release oxygen to control microbial growth in the mouth and reduce halitosis, e.g., hydrogen peroxide.

- *Analgesic agents*:
  Anti-inflammatory agents such as benzydamine hydrochloride inhibit inflammatory cytokines such as prostaglandins and may be used for the management discomfort associated with of oral ulcers and mucositis (see Chapter 12).

- *Miscellaneous agents*:
  Sodium chloride is one of the most cheap and effective agent to be used as a mouthwash (see Chapter 12).

11.3 FLUORIDE MOUTHWASHES

Fluoridated mouthwashes are recommended as an additional fluoride vehicle for some individuals with an increased risk of dental caries. As mentioned before, fluoridated mouthwashes are not a substitute for mechanical cleaning and use of a fluoridated toothpaste[2, 3]. Fluoride mouthwashes can be recommended for individuals with a high caries risk from the age of 6 years. However, there

Table 11.1 Common Regimens for Fluoride-Based Mouthwashes

Fluoride mouthwashes regimens[a]	Usage	Commercial preparations
Low potency/high frequency		
0.05% w/v sodium fluoride (~225 ppm F) equivalent to 500 µg/mL Alcohol-free	Daily use (once or twice per day)	FLUORIGARD® ACT® Anticavity
High potency/low frequency		
0.2% w/v sodium fluoride (900 ppm F) equivalent to 2 mg/mL Alcohol-free	Weekly use	PreviDent® Dental Rinse

[a] A rinse of 1–2 minutes is generally recommended.

are some variations in these recommendations in different countries[3, 4]. Swallowing reflexes must be in good function to avoid accidental swallowing, to help avoid detrimental side effects such as dental fluorosis in the growing child from chronic exposure. Common indications for fluoride mouthwash include:

- Xerostomia
- Active coronal and/or root surface caries
- Impaired ability to maintain oral hygiene
- Orthodontic appliances
- Prosthodontic appliances

Clinically, fluoridated mouthwashes are available as either low or high potency regimens, as summarised in Table 11.1.

11.4 ANTIMICROBIAL MOUTHWASHES

The main indications for antimicrobial mouthwashes include the following:

- Gingivitis (gingival bleeding)
- Halitosis
- Orthodontic appliances
- Prophylactic rinse prior to dental treatment
- Pre- and post-surgical interventions (oral surgery, periodontal surgery)
- *Systemic conditions*:
  - Physical or mental disability
  - Immunosuppressive conditions and therapy
  - Cytotoxic chemotherapy
  - Radiation therapy for head and neck cancer
  - Prevention/management medication-related osteonecrosis of jaws (see Chapter 16)

The most commonly used antimicrobial agents with evidence of clinical efficacy are discussed in the following text.

11.4.1 CHLORHEXIDINE

Chlorhexidine is a biguanide and marketed as a digluconate salt. It is the most common and effective chemical agent available for plaque control. There is evidence that chlorhexidine has a specific effect in inhibiting the formation of plaque on teeth. A chlorhexidine mouthwash may be useful as an adjunct to other oral hygiene measures or when tooth brushing is not possible.

Mechanism of action: Positively charged chlorhexidine molecule binds to negatively charged microbial cell wall and alters the cytoplasmic equilibrium of the bacterial cell resulting in leakage of potassium and phosphorus out of the cell with precipitation of the cytoplasmic contents and finally microbial cell death. It is effective against a variety of gram-negative and gram-positive bacteria, yeast etc.

Chlorhexidine derives its antiplaque efficacy from its ability to adhere to hydroxyapatite, dental pellicle, salivary glycoproteins and mucous membranes. Approximately, 30% of the active ingredient, chlorhexidine gluconate, is retained in the oral cavity following rinsing and subsequently released over an 8–12-hour period.

INDICATIONS FOR USE:

- *Indications for short-term use (2–4 weeks)*:

  Gingivitis, following periodontal surgery, following oral surgery, initial periodontal therapy and candidiasis.

- *Indications for intermittent use (alternating on and off every 1–2 months)*:

  Gingivitis, periodontal maintenance, physically and mentally handicapped, high caries activity and extensive prosthetic reconstruction.

- *Indications for long-term use (3 months or more)*:

  Impaired host resistance (AIDS, leukaemia, renal disease, bone marrow transplants, agranulocytosis and thrombocytopenia); physically handicapped (rheumatoid arthritis and scleroderma, etc.); cytotoxic and immunosuppressive drug therapy, radiation therapy; also, gingivitis, periodontal surgery, handicapped patients and orthodontic therapy.

  Side effects: *Tooth* staining and altered taste sensation though these are reduced at lower concentrations. It also increases calculus formation and may cause desquamation of oral mucosa. Parotid gland sialadenitis and tongue paraesthesia reported less frequently. There is also a risk of hypersensitivity and allergy; cases of fatal anaphylaxis are reported with chlorhexidine mouthwashes. Long-term use may lead to oral dysbiosis and contribute to antimicrobial resistance[5].

  Toxicity: Very low toxicity due to poor absorption from the GIT, 90% excreted in the faeces; there is no accumulation in the body and no harmful by-products are formed in the body.

  Cautions: It may stain composite restorations; avoid in pregnancy, breastfeeding, and under the age of 12 years.

COMMERCIAL CHLORHEXIDINE PREPARATIONS:

- *Corsodyl® original mouthwash* chlorhexidine digluconate 0.2% w/v; alcohol-free

- *PerioGard® oral rinse* chlorhexidine digluconate 0.12% w/v; alcohol-free

- *Corsodyl daily mouthwash* chlorhexidine digluconate 0.06% w/v with sodium fluoride (250 ppm F); alcohol-free

- *Kin* Gingival Complex mouthwash chlorhexidine digluconate 0.12% w/v; alcohol-free
  Kin Periokin mouthwash chlorhexidine digluconate 0.20% w/v; alcohol-free

DIRECTIONS FOR USE:

Rinse the mouth with 10 mL for 30–60 seconds and spit out. Do not mix with water. Used twice daily. Do not swallow and do not rinse with water. Do not eat or drink for at least 30 minutes after application. Do not drink from the bottle.

11.4.2 POVIDONE-IODINE

Povidone-iodine is a complex of iodine and povidone and following contact with oral tissues, it gradually releases free iodine which exhibits broad-spectrum antimicrobial activity against bacteria, fungi and viruses. Povidone-iodine mouthwash is useful for mucosal infections but does not inhibit plaque accumulation. It should not be used for period longer than 14 days since a significant amount of iodine is absorbed. There is no convincing evidence that gargles are effective.

It should be used with caution in pregnancy and breastfeeding. It is contra-indicated for regular use in patients with thyroid disorders or those receiving lithium therapy. Its side effects include idiosyncratic mucosal irritation and hypersensitivity reactions; may interfere with thyroid function tests and with tests for occult blood.

COMMERCIAL PREPARATIONS:

Betadine®

Mouthwash or gargle, povidone-iodine 1%.
Adults and children over 6 years, up to 10 mL undiluted or diluted with an equal quantity of warm water for up to 30 seconds up to 4 times daily for up to 14 days.

Following the COVID-19 pandemic, there has been a growing interest in the use of antimicrobial rinses containing chlorhexidine, povidone-iodine and hydrogen peroxide to reduce salivary load of SARS COV-2 virus and minimise its spread during aerosol-generating dental procedures[6]. Although prophylactic rinsing with antimicrobial mouthwashes may be helpful to reduce the viral load in saliva, further evidence is required to determine if such measures reduce the transmission of SARS COV-2 virus in dental settings[7].

11.4.3 DESENSITISING MOUTHWASHES

Mouthwashes containing an active desensitising agent are regarded as an adjunct method of treatment to patients suffering from dentine or root sensitivity. The underlying mechanisms of desensitising mouthwashes are similar to desensitising toothpastes which are summarised in Chapter 10 (Table 10.3).

Desensitising mouthwashes usually contain fluorides, potassium nitrate alone or in combination; additional products to seal the exposed dentinal tubules may be added such as arginine. Desensitising mouthwashes may offer variable degree of success, and generally in-office treatment of dentine sensitivity may offer rapid and more effective relief and is the preferred option for most patients.

COMMERCIAL PREPARATIONS:

Sensodyne® mouthwash cool mint:
  3% w/w potassium nitrate and 0.048% w/w sodium fluoride (217 ppm F)

Colgate® Sensitive Pro-Relief™ mouthwash:
  0.8% arginine copolymer and sodium fluoride (225 ppm F)

11.4.4 TOOTH WHITENING MOUTHWASHES

Mouthwashes with acclaimed tooth whitening ability are commercially available over-the-counter with variable active agents. Most common active ingredient is hydrogen peroxide (1.5–2%), a bleaching agent with a strong oxidising property. Other active agents include sodium peroxyborate, sodium hexametaphosphate and charcoal.

Despite claims by manufacturers, to date, the efficacy of whitening agents remains questionable, and therefore, no commercial preparations are recommended. Additionally, there are safety concerns with some of the products in whitening mouthwashes. Dry mouth, increased gum sensitivity and tooth staining have been reported following the use of charcoal-based mouthwashes.

Whitening and charcoal-based mouthwashes are only recommended for adults and children aged 12 years and above. Additionally, charcoal-based mouthwashes are not recommended for pregnant women[8].

11.4.5 HERBAL MOUTHWASHES

Mouthwashes based on various herbal products have recently been introduced and represent a promising therapeutic alternative.

Examples of herbal products added to mouthwashes include:

- *Aloe barbadensis* (*Aloe vera*)

- *Azadirachta indica* (Neem tree)

- *Camellia sinensis* (Green tea)

- *Glycyrrhiza glabra* (Liquorice)

- Propolis (Bees wax)

- Red ginseng (*Panax ginseng* plant)

- *Salvadora persica* (Miswak tree)

- *Zingiber officinale* (Ginger)

However, as with herbal toothpastes, further clinical evidence is required to support the routine use of herbal mouthwashes.

11.5 SUMMARY

Given the available evidence, a clear message to the patients must emphasise that mouthwashes should not be used to replace regular tooth brushing with a fluoridated toothpaste and use of interdental cleaning aids. Fluoride mouthwashes are recommended as an adjunct to standard oral hygiene measures for individuals with a high risk of caries. Mouthwashes with other active ingredients may be advised to patients depending on specific risks and clinical indication(s). Long-term use of alcohol-based mouthwashes and mouthwashes containing active antimicrobial agents should be discouraged due to the risk of side effects and adverse reactions.

RESOURCES

RESOURCES FOR DENTAL PROFESSIONALS

National Health Service. Chlorhexidine. https://www.nhs.uk/medicines/chlorhexidine.

Australian Commission on Safety and Quality in Health Care. www.nps.org.au/australian-prescriber/articles/mouthwashes (accessed February 2024).

RESOURCES FOR DENTAL PATIENTS

American Dental Association. https://www.mouthhealthy.org/en/all-topics-a-z/mouthwash (accessed February 2024).

Cleveland Clinic. Oral hygiene. https://my.clevelandclinic.org/health/diseases/16914-oral-hygiene (accessed February 2024).

REFERENCES

1. Poppolo, D.F. and Ouanounou, A. (2022). Chlorhexidine in dentistry: pharmacology, uses, and adverse effects. *International Dental Journal* 72: 269–277.

2. Marinho, V.C.C., Chong, L.Y., Worthington, H.V., and Walsh, T. (2016). Fluoride mouthrinses for preventing dental caries in children and adolescents. *Cochrane Database of Systematic Reviews* 7: CD002284.

3. Delivering Better Oral Health (2021). Chapter 13: Evidence base for recommendations in the summary guidance tables. https://www.gov.uk/government/publications/delivering-better-oral-health-an-evidence-based-toolkit-for-prevention/chapter-13-evidence-base-for-recommendations-in-the-summary-guidance-tables#fn:6 (accessed 5 May 2023).

4. Do, L. and Australian Research Centre for Population Oral Health (2020). Guidelines for use of fluorides in Australia: update 2019. *Australian Dental Journal* 65: 30–38.

5. Brookes, Z.L.S., Bescos, R., Belfield, L.A. et al. (2020). Current uses of chlorhexidine for management of oral disease: a narrative review. *Journal of Dentistry* 103: 103497. https://doi.org/10.1016/j.jdent.2020.103497.

6. Chaudhary, P., Melkonyan, A., Meethil, A. et al. (2021). Estimating salivary carriage of severe acute respiratory syndrome coronavirus 2 in nonsymptomatic people and efficacy of mouthrinse in reducing viral load: a randomized controlled trial. *Journal of the American Dental Association* 152 (11): 903–908. https://doi.org/10.1016/j.adaj.2021.05.021.

7. Ali, K. and Raja, M. (2020). Coronavirus disease 2019 (COVID-19): challenges and management of aerosol-generating procedures in dentistry. *Evidence-Based Dentistry* 21 (2): 44–45.

8. Brooks, J.K., Bashirelahi, N., Hsia, R.-C., and Reynolds, M.A. (2020). Charcoal-based mouthwashes: a literature review. *British Dental Journal* 228: 290–294.

Agents Used in the Management of Oral Ulceration

CHAPTER 12

Kamran Ali

Qatar University, QU Health, College of Dental Medicine, Doha, Qatar

12.1 INTRODUCTION

Oral ulcers constitute one of the commonest oral mucosal pathologies encountered in dental practice[1, 2]. Oral ulceration may result from local causes such as trauma or may be indicative of an underlying systemic disorder, or be linked to drug usage. Recurrent aphthous ulcers (RAUs) are the commonest type of oral ulcers[3, 4]. More importantly, oral mucosal ulceration could be related to malignancy such as oral squamous cell carcinoma[5]. Therefore, it is important that dentists and dental care professionals to recognise different types of oral ulcers for appropriate management including timely referral to specialists when indicated[6]. Table 12.1 summarises the common local and systemic causes of oral ulceration[7]. Drug-associated oral ulcerations (DAOUs) are summarised in Table 12.2.

Although the focus of the present chapter is on DAOU (discussed later), patients taking medications are not exempt from ulceration from other causes summarised in Table 12.1. The following points may be helpful to recognise and manage patients presenting with oral ulcers.

- Oral ulcers may result from physical trauma from hot food, sharp edges of teeth, and dental appliances such as dentures, removable orthodontic appliances or loose orthodontic wires, and bands. It is important to rule out local trauma to the oral mucosa before considering other causes of oral ulceration.

- RAUs are common, and anaemia is a recognised risk factor for RAU. Although local pain relief using appropriate measures is essential, it is important for the dental professionals to consult with the patient's medical physician to request haematological investigations, including complete blood count, serum ferritin, folate and vitamin B_{12} levels. Medical referral allows a more holistic patient management and may help identify or rule out underlying anaemia as a risk factor for RAUs.

- Oral ulcers secondary to infections may be associated with systemic signs and symptoms such as fever, malaise, anorexia, lymphadenopathy and other specific manifestations of infection.

- Oral ulcers may also be related to malignancy. Oral squamous cell carcinoma (OSCC) may present as a non-healing ulcer (Figure 12.1). It is important to note that oral ulceration caused by OSCC is usually painless and may give a false sense of self-reassurance to patients leading to a delay in seeking professional advice. Pain may be associated with secondary infection of

Clinical Dental Pharmacology, First Edition. Edited by Kamran Ali.
© 2024 John Wiley & Sons Ltd. Published 2024 by John Wiley & Sons Ltd.

ulceration caused by OSCC or may result from extensive tissue invasion and involvement of local nerves (late sign). Rarely, oral ulceration may develop as a manifestation of other types of malignancies such as non-Hodgkin's lymphoma (Figure 12.2) or metastatic cancers. Oral ulcers which persist for more than 3 weeks and cannot be attributed to a local or systemic cause should raise a suspicion of OSCC, and an urgent referral to an oral and maxillofacial surgeon should be made for an expert opinion.

Table 12.1 Differential Diagnosis of Oral Ulceration

Cause	Examples
Traumatic	Mechanical, chemical, thermal, electric, radiation
Recurrent aphthae	Minor, major and herpetiform
Infection	
Bacterial	Necrotising periodontal diseases; scarlet fever; syphilis; tuberculosis; diphtheria; cancrum oris
Viral	Herpes simplex, Varicella Zoster; Herpangina. Hand foot and mouth disease
Fungal	Mucormycosis; cryptococcosis; histoplasmosis; aspergillosis; paracoccidiomycosis
Protozoal	Leishmaniasis
Neoplastic	Squamous cell carcinoma (Figure 12.1), non-Hodgkin lymphoma (Figure 12.2), metastatic cancers
Haematological disorders	Anaemia; leukaemia; neutropenia; hyper-eosinophilic syndrome
GIT diseases	Coeliac disease; Crohn's disease; ulcerative colitis
Mucocutaneous diseases	Erosive lichen planus; pemphigus vulgaris; mucous membrane pemphigoid; bullous pemphigoid; linear IgA disease; erythema multiforme; Reiter's disease; Bechet's syndrome; epidermolysis bullosa
Connective tissue diseases	Lupus erythematosus; periarteritis nodosa; giant cell arteritis

Table 12.2 Drugs Associated with Oral Ulcers

Drug type	Examples
Angiotensin-converting enzyme (ACE) inhibitors	Captopril
Angiotensin-II receptor antagonist	Losartan
Antiarrhythmic drugs	Disopyramide, quinidine
Antibiotics	Sulphonamides, vancomycin, aztreonam
Anticholinergics	Emepronium
Anticoagulants	Phenindione, warfarin
Antiepileptics	Phenytoin, carbamazepine
Antifungal drugs	Fluconazole
Antigout drugs	Allopurinol
Antimalarials	Proguanil
Antiparasitic drugs	Levamisole

Table 12.2 (Continued)

Drug type	Examples
Antipsychotics	Olanzapine, sertraline; quetiapine
Antiretroviral drugs	Indinavir, zalcitabine
Antirheumatic drugs	Gold, penicillamine
Antithyroid drugs	Methimazole, propylthiouracil
Antiresorptive drugs	Bisphosphonates, e.g., alendronic acid
	RANKL inhibitors, e.g., denosumab
Cytotoxic drugs	Bleomycin, hydroxyurea, doxorubicin, vincristine, chlorambucil, carboplatin, cisplatin, cytarabines, melphalan, methotrexate
Immuno-modulating drugs	Interferons, molgramostim
Immunosuppressive drugs	Cyclosporine, azathioprine, tacrolimus, everolimus, adalimumab
Non-steroidal anti-inflammatory drugs (NSAIDs)	Indomethacin, diclofenac, sulindac, naproxen, phenylbutazone, ketorolac
Selective serotonin release inhibitors (SSRIs)	Sertraline, fluoxetine
Statins	Atorvastatin
Steroids	Flunisolide
Vasodilators	Nicorandil
β-receptor agonists	Isoprenaline, terbutaline
Miscellaneous	Pancreatin
	Potassium chloride

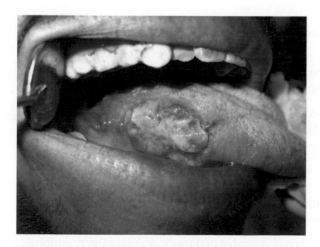

FIGURE 12.1 A large nodulo-ulcerative growth on the right lateral border of the tongue. This lesion was diagnosed as a squamous cell carcinoma

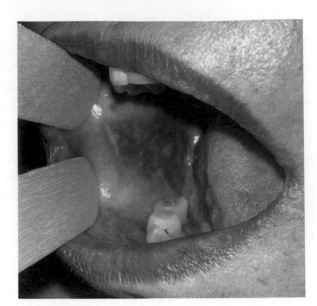

FIGURE 12.2   Erythema and ulceration on the right buccal mucosa in a patient diagnosed with non-Hodgkin's lymphoma

12.2 DRUG-ASSOCIATED ORAL ULCERS (DAOUs)

DAOUs may represent exacerbation of existing aphthous ulcers or lichenoid reactions or may be specifically related to adverse effects of medications[8–10]. While it is difficult to include every single drug which may be associated with development and/or exacerbation of oral ulcerations, common examples are summarised in Table 12.2.

12.2.1 PRINCIPLES OF DIAGNOSIS

- Review medical history including all prescribed/non-prescribed medications and nutritional supplements.

- Common causes of oral ulceration need to be excluded for, e.g., trauma, aphthae, infections, post-irradiation and ulcers related to systemic disorders (see Table 12.1).

- Request the patient's physician for a complete blood count to rule out anaemia (common risk factor for aphthous oral ulceration) and to identify other haematological abnormalities.

- For DAOUs, determine if the appearance of oral ulcers coincides with starting any new medication(s). If a patient presents with oral ulcers (or other signs potentially associated with oral side effects of drugs) review adverse reactions of all medications consumed by the patient using an authentic source such as the British National Formulary (BNF) or patient information leaflets (PILs) provided by the manufacturer.

- Additional investigations may be undertaken in specialist oral medicine/oral surgery settings:
  - Consider culture and sensitivity using oral swab samples to rule out infection.
  - Consider exfoliative cytology to determine the nature of the ulcer. This is particularly important if there is a suspicion of malignancy and in cases which are difficult to diagnose clinically.
  - Consider performing a biopsy for persistent, non-healing lesions especially in patients with risk factors for OSCC, e.g., smoking, alcohol, human papilloma virus (HPV) infection.

12.2.2 PRINCIPLES OF TREATMENT

The definitive management should be directed at eliminating/addressing the underlying cause of ulceration. Suspected DAOUs require consultation with prescribing medical physician/specialist to discuss if the medication responsible for oral ulceration can be changed with a suitable alternative.

Dentists may provide symptomatic treatment for painful oral ulcers associated with inflammation[11]. It is important to rule out drug allergy to the relevant medication and consider patient's medical history and concurrent medications to minimise side effects and drug interactions. Common measures to reduce pain and inflammation associated with oral ulcers include the following:

- *Mouthwashes*:
  - Saline rinses (half a teaspoon of salt mixed in a glass of warm water) 4–6 hourly until healing is achieved: spit after rinsing.
  - Chlorhexidine mouthwash 0.2%; rinse mouth with 10 mL for 1 minute twice daily until healing is achieved; spit out the mouthwash, do not swallow.
  - Hydrogen peroxide mouthwash 6%; rinse mouth with 15 mL in half a glass of water for 2–3 minutes 8-hourly until healing is achieved; spit out the mouthwash, do not swallow.

- *Topical analgesics*:
  - Benzydamine mouthwash 0.15%; 15 mL every 90 minutes; spit out the mouthwash after rinsing. Can be used for up to 7 days.
  - Benzydamine oro-mucosal spray 0.15%; four sprays on affected site every 90 minutes.

- *Topical anaesthetics*:
  - Lidocaine 5% ointment.
  - Lidocaine 10% or 15% aerosol spray.
  - Benzocaine 20% gel.

- *Topical antiseptics*:
  - Chlorhexidine gluconate gel 1%.

- *Topical antibiotics*:
  - Doxycycline 100 mg dispersible tablets, 1 tablet dissolved in 180 mL of water; rinse for 2 minutes 4 times daily for 3 days; do not swallow.

- *Topical corticosteroids*:
  - Beclometasone CFC-free inhaler 50 μg/metred dose (Qvar®; Clenil Modulite®); 1–2 puffs directed on the lesion twice daily.
  - Betamethasone soluble tablets 500 μg: 1 tablet dissolved in 10 mL water and used as a mouthwash 4 times/day; do not swallow.
  - Hydrocortisone oro-mucosal tablets 2.5 mg: 1 tablet dissolved adjacent to the ulcer 4 times/day.

- *Referral to a specialist*:
  - If ulcers appear to be related to a systemic medication, liaise with the prescribing physician to discuss the options of a suitable replacement medication.
  - The risk of immunosuppression should be considered when prescribing steroid preparations and medical advice may be sought if required.
  - Referral to a specialist in oral medicine is advised if the oral ulcers are persistent or refractory to symptomatic management.

- Urgent referral to an oral and maxillofacial surgeon should be made if there is a suspicion that ulceration may be related to a malignancy, especially if risk factors related to oral cancer are present, i.e., smoking or alcohol.

ACKNOWLEDGEMENTS

Figure 12.2 provided by Dr Gulraiz Zulfiqar, Jinnah Hospital, Lahore Pakistan.

RESOURCES

RESOURCES FOR DENTAL PROFESSIONALS

Scottish Clinical Dental Effectiveness Programme (SDCEP). Management of acute dental problems. http://madp.sdcep.org.uk (accessed 23 February 2024).

RESOURCES FOR DENTAL PATIENTS

Mayo Clinic. CANKER sore. https://www.mayoclinic.org/diseases-conditions/canker-sore/symptoms-causes/syc-20370615 (accessed 25 February 2024).

REFERENCES

1. Yousefi, H. and Abdollahi, M. (2019). An update on drug-induced oral reactions. *Journal of Pharmacy and Pharmaceutical Sciences* 21: 171–183.

2. Field, E.A. and Allan, R.B. (2003). Review article: oral ulceration - aetiopathogenesis, clinical diagnosis and management in the gastrointestinal clinic. *Alimentary Pharmacology and Therapeutics* 18: 949–962. https://doi.org/10.1046/j.1365-2036.2003.01782.x.

3. Minhas, S., Sajjad, A., Kashif, M. et al. (2019). Oral ulcers presentation in systemic diseases: an update. *Open Access Macedonian Journal of Medical Sciences* 7: 3341.

4. Scully, C. and Porter, S. (2008). Oral mucosal disease: recurrent aphthous stomatitis. *British Journal of Oral and Maxillofacial Surgery* 46: 198–206.

5. Bagan, J., Sarrion, G., and Jimenez, Y. (2010). Oral cancer: clinical features. *Oral Oncology* 46: 414–417.

6. Teoh, L., Moses, G., and McCullough, M.J. (2019). A review and guide to drug-associated oral adverse effects—Oral mucosal and lichenoid reactions. Part 2. *Journal of Oral Pathology and Medicine* 48: 637–646.

7. Lehman, J.S. and Rogers, R.S. III, (2016). Acute oral ulcers. *Clinics in Dermatology* 34: 470–474.

8. Porter, S.R. and Scully, C. (2000). Adverse drug reactions in the mouth. *Clinics in Dermatology* 18: 525–532. https://doi.org/10.1016/S0738-081X(00)00143-7.

9. Scully, C. and Bagan, J.V. (2004). Adverse drug reactions in the orofacial region. *Critical Reviews in Oral Biology and Medicine* 15: 221–239. https://doi.org/10.1177/154411130401500405.

10. Ali, K., Raja, M., Osman, S. et al. (2022). Recognition and management of drug-associated oral ulceration: a review. *British Dental Journal* 233: 564–568.

11. Mashrah, M.A., Fang, Y., Song, W. et al. (2023). Topical medications for the treatment of recurrent aphthous stomatitis: a network meta-analysis. *Journal of Oral Pathology & Medicine* 52: 811–825. https://doi.org/10.1111/jop.13480.

Agents Used in the Management of Xerostomia

CHAPTER 13

Mahwish Raja

Qatar University, QU Health, College of Dental Medicine, Doha, Qatar

13.1 INTRODUCTION

Xerostomia (zee·ruh·stow·mee·uh) or dry mouth is a clinical manifestation of salivary gland dysfunction but does not in itself represent a specific disease. Xerostomia may be temporary or permanent depending on the specific cause and its duration[1]. Temporary or transient xerostomia while quite disconcerting to the patient seldom produces notable changes in the oral mucosa. On the other hand, long-standing xerostomia may be associated with numerous complications[2]. The common causes of xerostomia are summarised in Table 13.1.

CLINICAL PRESENTATION:
All degrees of xerostomia exist, i.e., from mild to severe.

(a) Mild xerostomia may result in a dry or burning sensation, but the mucosa appears normal.

(b) Moderate to severe xerostomia may lead to extreme discomfort and soreness with changes in oral mucosa including:
   - Inflammation with a tendency for accumulation of debris.
   - Atrophy of the lingual papillae, inflammation, fissuring, cracking and areas of denudation.
   - Crackling of the lips and fissuring of the corners of the mouth.

COMPLICATIONS:

(a) Severe discomfort and psychological disturbances.

(b) High risk of dental caries and subsequent loss of teeth.

(c) Periodontal disease.

(d) Taste disturbances.

(e) Difficulty in wearing artificial dentures and other dental prostheses.

(f) Oral candidiasis.

   Oral complications of xerostomia can adversely affect the patient's dietary intake, general health and quality of life[3, 4].

13.2 MANAGEMENT OF XEROSTOMIA

The most important aspect of treatment is accurate diagnosis. It is extremely important to determine the exact cause of xerostomia with the aid of a thorough history and clinical examination. Patients may require additional investigations such as sialometry, salivary gland imaging,

Clinical Dental Pharmacology, First Edition. Edited by Kamran Ali.
© 2024 John Wiley & Sons Ltd. Published 2024 by John Wiley & Sons Ltd.

Table 13.1   Causes of Xerostomia

- Emotional reaction (temporary)
- Dehydration
  - Vomiting
  - Diarrhoea
  - Blood loss
  - Diabetes mellitus
  - Diabetes insipidus
- Salivary gland infections (usually temporary)
- Radiation therapy for head and neck cancers
- Sjögren's syndrome
- Sialolithiasis (salivary duct stones)
- Developmental: Salivary gland aplasia or atresia of salivary duct
- Drugs
  - Antihistamines, e.g., cetirizine, cyclizine, loratadine, ketotifen
  - Anti-depressants, e.g., sertraline, fluoxetine, mirtazapine, citalopram
  - Anti-muscarinics, e.g., atropine
  - Anti-psychotics, e.g., olanzapine, chlorpromazine, risperidone
  - Benzodiazepines, e.g., diazepam, midazolam
  - Diuretics, e.g., furosemide
  - Immunomodulators, e.g., interferon
  - Mono amino-oxidase (MAO) inhibitors, e.g., selegiline
  - Opioids, e.g., morphine, dihydrocodeine, buprenorphine
  - Recreational drugs, e.g., ecstasy, cannabis
  - *Serotonin 5-HT-receptor agonists,* e.g.*, rizatriptan*
  - Tricyclic antidepressants, e.g., amitriptyline, nortriptyline, clomipramine, doxepin

biopsy and haematological investigations to establish a definitive diagnosis and this can be best achieved through specialist referral.

Although there are numerous potential causes of xerostomia, a careful medical history can often help identify the most likely cause in a given patient. The following strategies may be helpful to determine the cause of xerostomia:

- Given that xerostomia may be associated with a large number of prescription and non-prescription drugs, drug-induced xerostomia is the most common cause and a review of patient's medications may allow dentists to identify a causative agent. Apart from recognising common medications-associated xerostomia (Table 13.1), it is advisable to review the side effects of all medications used by a patient by using an appropriate professional resource or the patient information leaflets accompanying prescribed medications.

- Chronic dehydration may be related to underlying medical disorders such as diabetes mellitus. Suboptimal blood glucose control may result in excessive urination (polyuria) due to osmotic diuresis, and understandably this leads to dehydration and increased thirst (polydipsia).

- A combination of xerostomia and xerophthalmia (dry eyes) may be suggestive of Sjögren's syndrome. The symptoms may occur in isolation (primary Sjögren's syndrome) or secondary to an underlying autoimmune disorder (secondary) Sjögren's syndrome. Definitive diagnosis requires appropriate investigations (e.g., serum auto-antibody profile and salivary gland biopsy) in specialist settings. Specialist referral of patients with Sjögren's syndrome is also important due to an elevated risk of salivary gland lymphoma. Therefore, these patients should be under long-term care of specialists to monitor clinical and laboratory markers associated with an increased risk of salivary gland lymphoma.

- Xerostomia may be severe in patients who receive radiotherapy for head and neck cancers. Such patients are already made aware during their preparation and consent for radiotherapy that xerostomia is a complication of radiation-induced damage to the salivary glands. While cancer patients are managed in specialist hospital settings, it is not unusual for dentists to provide oral care to these patients. Therefore, dentists in general practice settings should be able to provide symptomatic management of radiation-induced xerostomia.

Identification of an underlying cause of xerostomia is required to plan the course of treatment. Obviously if the underlying cause of xerostomia can be discovered, it should be managed appropriately by liaising with medical colleagues. In any case, dentists should be able to provide symptomatic relief to patients presenting with xerostomia. Moreover, appropriate measures should be taken to provide oral care. The focus should be prevention and management of oral complications secondary to xerostomia including dental caries, and periodontal disease to avoid premature tooth loss[2].

13.2.1 GENERAL MEASURES

- Advise the patients to stay well hydrated throughout the day.
  - Consider drinking milk at mealtimes as the fats in the milk can improve moisturising the mucosa and aid in swallowing.
  - Use appropriate lip moisturisers (e.g., lanolin-based products) to prevent dryness and crackling.
  - Use a cool air humidifier in the bedroom especially during the night.
  - Seek medical advice to control mouth breathing and snoring.

  The following may worsen xerostomia and should be avoided:
- Caffeine, smoking and alcohol including alcohol-containing mouthwashes.
- Foods and beverages with a high acid or sugar content.
- Dry, hard-to-chew foods.
- Gums, candies, oral care products and other medications that contain sugars, consider using sugar-free products.

13.2.2 MEDICATION-INDUCED XEROSTOMIA

Medication-induced xerostomia is common and may be caused by hundreds of medications including over-the-counter drugs for common ailments[5]. If a medication is the suspected cause of xerostomia, consult with the patient's physician to discuss alternate options, reducing the dosage and/or modifying the frequency and timing of the medication.

13.2.3 ORAL AND DENTAL CARE

Maintenance of a meticulous oral hygiene is critical in patients with xerostomia due to the high risk of dental caries and oral infections[6].

- Dentate patients must brush their teeth twice daily with fluoride-containing toothpaste and use appropriate interdental cleaning aids, e.g., dental floss/interdental brushes; may also need a prescription of a daily use fluoride gel (0.4% stannous fluoride and 1.0% sodium fluoride) or an appropriate fluoride mouthwash to prevent dental decay.
  - Patients with severe xerostomia may be prescribed high-fluoride toothpastes such as sodium fluoride toothpaste 0.619% (2800 ppm) or sodium fluoride toothpaste 1.1% (5000 ppm) to be used 2–3 times each day, respectively (Chapter 10).
  - Sodium fluoride toothpaste 0.05%; rinse with 10 mL for 1 minute and spit out; do not swallow.
  - Six monthly dental visits with yearly bitewings.

- Edentulous patients wearing dentures must maintain an excellent denture hygiene.

- Prompt management of oral candidiasis and other opportunistic infections.

13.2.4 SALIVARY STIMULANTS

These will only be helpful where there is some glandular activity present and the following agents have been used:

(i) Use sugar-free (xylitol-based) salivary stimulants such as chewing gum and sucking ice, sugar-free fruit pastilles, etc.

(ii) Mouth lubricants and lemon mucilage (for edentulous patients only).

13.2.5 SALIVARY SUBSTITUTES/ORAL MOISTURISERS (ARTIFICIAL SALIVA)

Although not a cure, artificial saliva can provide symptomatic relief of dry mouth and improve the quality of life. Some artificial salivary preparations are available over the counter, while others require a prescription. Typical ingredients include carboxymethylcellulose and glycerine (to increase viscosity); buffering and flavouring agents (e.g., sorbitol, xylitol), and calcium and phosphate and fluoride ions. However, artificial saliva products do not contain the digestive and antibacterial enzymes or other proteins of biological saliva. A balanced artificial saliva should be of a neutral pH and contain electrolytes (including fluoride) to correspond to the composition of saliva.

Some common products include:

- *Saliva Orthana®* (Porcine source): Available as oral spray 50 mL and lozenges

- *Biotene® Oralbalance* (Animal source): *Saliva replacement gel 50* g

- *Glandosane®* (Non-animal source): Aerosol spray 50 mL (natural, peppermint and lemon flavours)

- *Saliveze®* (Non-animal source): *Oral spray 50* mL

- *Xerotin®* (Non-animal source): *Oral spray 100* mL

- NeutraSal® (Supersaturated calcium phosphate): Available as powder for reconstitution with water and used as a mouth rinse – do not swallow. Requires a prescription

13.2.6 SYSTEMIC TREATMENT

Systemic treatment of xerostomia is based on cholinergic agents such as pilocarpine or cevimeline which enhance parasympathetic stimulation of salivary glands. They are reserved for patients with severe xerostomia such as following radiation therapy or Sjogren's syndrome and require a prescription[3, 7]. They are effective only in patients who have some residual salivary gland function and should be withdrawn if there is no response. Usually, these medications are prescribed by specialists in oral medicine and oral surgery.

Pilocarpine Hydrochloride Tablets (Salagen®)

Available as pilocarpine hydrochloride 5 mg oral tablets. The usual dose is 5 mg 3 times daily with or immediately after meals (last dose always with evening meal); maximum dose 30 mg daily.

Side effects: Sweating; also, chills, diarrhoea, nausea, vomiting, lacrimation, abdominal pain, amblyopia, hypertension, constipation, abnormal vision (see counselling), dizziness, rhinitis, asthenia, increased urinary frequency, headache, dyspepsia, vasodilatation, flushing may be encountered. Other possible side effects include respiratory distress, gastrointestinal spasm, AV block, tachycardia, bradycardia, other arrhythmias, hypotension, shock, confusion and tremors.

Contra-indications: Uncontrolled asthma and chronic obstructive airways disease (increased bronchial secretions and increased airways resistance); acute iritis, narrow-angle glaucoma; pregnancy and breastfeeding.

Counselling: Blurred vision may affect ability to drive, particularly at night, and to perform hazardous activities in reduced lighting.

Cevimeline Hydrochloride Capsules (Evoxac®)

Available as cevimeline hydrochloride capsules 30 mg; usual dose is 30 mg capsule 3 times a day.

Side effects: Headache, tiredness, hoarseness or loss of voice, bladder pain, frequent urge to urinate, painful urination, bloody or cloudy urine, body aches or pain, chills, breathing difficulties, ear and nasal congestion, vision changes, soft tissue bleeding.

Contra indications: Iritis, closed-angle glaucoma, angina, cardiac arrhythmias, asthma, chronic bronchitis, chronic obstructive pulmonary disease (COPD), cholecystitis, gall stones and renal stones.

13.3 SUMMARY

Although xerostomia may result from a variety of causes, drug-induced xerostomia is common. The most likely cause can often be identified with a careful medical history. Definitive diagnosis may require specialist referral. Dentists should be able to advise patients on appropriate measures to gain symptomatic relief with salivary stimulants, salivary substitutes and less commonly with prescription of systemic medications, as appropriate. Moreover, dentists should institute preventive measures to reduce the risk of dental caries and periodontal disease. These should include patient education on maintenance of meticulous oral hygiene, diet advice and home-based/in-office fluorides.

RESOURCES

RESOURCES FOR DENTAL PROFESSIONALS

ADA (American Dental Association). https://www.ada.org/resources/research/science-and-research-institute/oral-health-topics/xerostomia (accessed 23 February 2024).

RESOURCES FOR DENTAL PATIENTS

Mayo Clinic. https://www.mayoclinic.org/diseases-conditions/dry-mouth/symptoms-causes/syc-20356048 (accessed 23 February 2024).

REFERENCES

1. Tschoppe, P., Wolgin, M., Pischon, N., and Kielbassa, A.M. (2010). Etiologic factors of hyposalivation and consequences for oral health. *Quintessence International* 41 (4): 321–333.

2. Turner, M.D. (2016). Hyposalivation and xerostomia. Etiology, complications, and medical management. *Dental Clinics of North America* 60: 435–443.

3. Barbe, A.G., Schmidt, P., Bussmann, M. et al. (2018). Xerostomia and hyposalivation in orthogeriatric patients with fall history and impact on oral health-related quality of life. *Clinical Interventions in Aging* 13: 1971–1979.

4. Choi, J.H., Kim, M.J., and Kho, H.S. (2021). Oral health-related quality of life and associated factors

in patients with xerostomia. *International Journal of Dental Hygiene* 19 (3): 313–322.

5. Barbe, A.G. (2018). Medication-induced xerostomia and hyposalivation in the elderly: culprits, complications, and management. *Drugs & Aging* 35 (10): 877–885.

6. Deng, J., Jackson, L., Epstein, J.B. et al. (2015). Dental demineralization and caries in patients with head and neck cancer. *Oral Oncology* 51: 824–831.

7. Garg, A.K. and Malo, M. (1997). Manifestations and treatment of xerostomia and associated oral effects secondary to head and neck radiation therapy. *Journal of the American Dental Association* 128 (8): 1128–1133.

Systemic Medications

Systemic
Medications

SECTION 4

Oral Side Effects of Systemic Medications

CHAPTER 14

Kamran Ali

Qatar University, QU Health, College of Dental Medicine, Doha, Qatar

14.1 INTRODUCTION

Globally, an increasing number of people are prescribed drugs for underlying medical conditions. This increase in prescribed medications can be attributed to several factors such as population growth, improved life expectancy, better medical diagnosis, and a higher incidence of chronic conditions including hypertension, diabetes mellitus, and ischemic heart disease. In the United States, approximately 4.8 billion drug prescriptions were dispensed in 2022, while in England, the figure is over 1 billion, and this number is increasing annually[1, 2]. As a result of the rising number of people using prescribed medications, an increasing number of patients are experiencing oral complications in dental practices. Some patients may not link these complications to their medication(s) and may consult a dentist instead of their medical physician.

Patients use a vast array of systemic medications, and dentists may not always be completely familiar with the potential side effects of each drug. The frequent introduction of new medications in the market further exacerbates this issue. In addition, due to time constraints in clinical settings, dentists may not have sufficient time to associate oral signs and symptoms with the use of systemic medications. These factors can result in an incorrect diagnosis, and management may be limited to providing symptomatic relief only rather than identifying the underlying cause.

The following strategies are recommended when dentists encounter oral signs and symptoms which may be potentially related to patient's medications:

- Rule out drug involvement by identifying the potential side effects of patient's medications using authentic online resources and/or referring to the patient information leaflets (PILs) accompanying the individual medications being used by the patient.

- Seek advice from the medical colleagues who have prescribed the medications with suspected oral side effects, and it may be possible to replace such medications with suitable alternatives.

- Report adverse drug reactions (known or previously unrecognised) relevant authorities in the country where a dentist is practising. For example, in the United Kingdom, adverse drug reactions can be reported to the Medicines and Healthcare products Regulatory Agency (MHRA) while in the United States, these should be reported to the Food and Drug Administration (FDA).

14.2 DRUG-ASSOCIATED REACTIONS IN THE ORO-FACIAL REGION

A variety of side effects may manifest in the oro-facial region in patients using prescribed medications[3]. The most recognised and common oral side effects of medications are as follows:

Clinical Dental Pharmacology, First Edition. Edited by Kamran Ali.
© 2024 John Wiley & Sons Ltd. Published 2024 by John Wiley & Sons Ltd.

14.2.1 XEROSTOMIA

Drug-associated xerostomia is common, may be seen in patients taking a wide variety of medications including antihistamines, decongestants, antihypertensives, tricyclic antidepressants, and antipsychotic, and *parasympatholytic* drugs. These are discussed in more details in Chapter 13.

14.2.2 GINGIVAL OVERGROWTH

Gingival overgrowth is a well-recognised side effect of systemic medications and may be associated with long-term use of the following medications:

- Calcium channel blockers (CCBs) are used for the management of hypertension, angina pectoris and some cardiac arrhythmias. CCBs associated with gingival hyperplasia include nifedipine, nicardipine, manidipine, nisoldipine, cilnidipine, lacidipine, verapamil, diltiazem, amlodipine and felodipine.

- Immunosuppressive drugs such as basiliximab and cyclosporin

- Oral contraceptive agents.

- Phenytoin (formerly known as diphenylhydantoin), an anticonvulsant drug.

Severe gingival growth can be disfiguring (Figure 14.1) and can interfere with mastication and speech. Initially, this side effect can be discussed with the prescribing medical physician to evaluate if the medication responsible gingival overgrowth can be replaced with a suitable alternative. Local measures to improve oral hygiene and professional cleaning may help reduce inflammation in gingival tissues. The magnitude of benefits from local measures may vary. Surgical correction of gingival overgrowth remains to most popular option. This may be achieved with a conventional surgical scalpel, electrocautery or laser surgery.

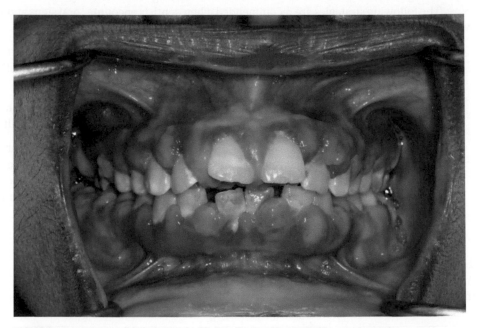

FIGURE 14.1   Generalised gingival enlargement in a patient taking cyclosporin

14.2.3 LICHENOID REACTIONS

Oral lichenoid reactions simulate classic lichen planus and may be associated with a wide variety of medications[4]. Some key examples include the following:

- Antibiotics, e.g., penicillins, metronidazole, tetracycline, streptomycin and *para*-amino salicylic acid

- Angiotensin-converting enzyme (ACE) inhibitors, e.g., captopril
  - CCBs, e.g., amlodipine (see Figure 14.2), nifedipine and felodipine

- Antithyroid agents, e.g., carbimazole

- Antigout agents, e.g., allopurinol

- Antimalarial agents, e.g., quinine, quinidine, chloroquine

- Antifungal agents, e.g., ketoconazole

- Anticonvulsants, e.g., carbamazepine, phenytoin

- Benzodiazepines, e.g., lorazepam

- Antiplatelet agents, e.g., dipyridamole

- Antirheumatic agents, e.g., gold, penicillamine

- Non-steroidal anti-inflammatory drugs, e.g., rofecoxib

- Oral hypoglycaemics, e.g., metformin

- Beta blockers, e.g., propranolol

- Phenothiazines, e.g., serentil

Lichenoid reactions simulate classical lichen planus. If association with medication can be identified, the dentist may be able to liaise with the prescribing medical physician to replace the

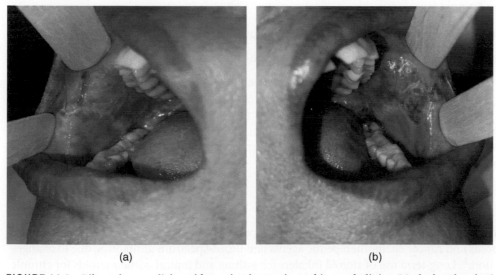

(a)   (b)

FIGURE 14.2   Bilateral severe lichenoid reaction in a patient taking amlodipine. Marked oral melanin pigmentation can also be noted

offending medication with a suitable alternative to achieve resolution. Symptomatic relief may be required for lesions associated with oral ulceration and pain using local measures described in Chapter 12.

Lichenoid reactions may be observed on oral mucosa adjacent to dental amalgam restorations. Replacement of amalgam fillings with a suitable material such as composite can help achieve resolution.

14.2.4 ALLERGIC AND HYPERSENSITIVITY REACTIONS

Hypersensitivity and allergic reactions may be associated with a large number of drugs, and any prior history must be confirmed with each patient. The most commonly implicated group of drugs include:

- Antibiotics, e.g., penicilins, cephalosporins and macrolides

- Local anaesthetics especially ester type, e.g., benzocaine

- Topical agents, e.g., chlorhexidine

Allergic and hypersensitivity reactions to drugs can range from mild, localised skin reactions to severe, systemic reactions that can be potentially life-threatening such as acute anaphylaxis (see Chapter 17). Although some patients may report common gastrointestinal side effects associated with various medications as 'allergy', patients concerns should always be taken seriously and the suspected medicine is best avoided.

14.2.5 ANGIOOEDEMA

Angioedema is characterised by rapid and marked swelling of the deeper layers of the skin and often involves the tissues around the eyes and lips. It can also affect the hands, feet and genitalia. Like other allergic and hypersensitivity reactions, angioedema may be triggered by drugs including the following:

- ACE inhibitors, e.g., enalapril

- Non-steroidal anti-inflammatory drugs, e.g., ibuprofen, naproxen

- Antibiotics, e.g., sulphonamides, clindamycin, co-trimoxazole and streptomycin

- Antifungal agents, e.g., ketoconazole, miconazole

- Anticonvulsants, e.g., carbamazepine

In addition, contact with latex products, e.g., gloves, suction tubes, etc. can also trigger angioedema. As with drug allergies, avoidance of suspected drugs and materials remains the most appropriate approach to prevention.

14.2.6 OPPORTUNISTIC ORAL INFECTIONS

Opportunistic oral infections may be encountered in patients on immunosuppressive drugs, including steroids and cancer chemotherapeutic agents and broad-spectrum antibiotics, due to changes in oral flora[5]. Long-term use of steroid inhalers for asthma and topical corticosteroids for chronic oral mucosal conditions such as erosive lichen planus can also increase the risk of opportunistic oral infections. Moreover, xerostomia is also a risk factor for opportunistic oral infections, and sometimes xerostomia itself may be induced by drugs (see Chapter 13). Oral candidiasis is the one the most recognised opportunistic infection in the mouth. Pseudomembranous candidiasis (oral thrush) and acute atrophic candidiasis (antibiotic sore mouth) are well-recognised forms of oral candidiasis associated with drug use (see Chapter 9). In addition, reactivation of oral herpes viruses can be associated with immunosuppression (see Chapter 8).

14.2.7 TOOTH DISCOLOURATION

Tooth discolouration may result from the use of the following:

- Antibiotics, e.g., tetracyclines, clarithromycin, metronidazole
- ACE inhibitors, e.g., lisinopril
- Antimicrobial agents, e.g., chlorhexidine
- Fluorides
- Iron therapy

Tetracycline-induced tooth discoloration is a side effect that occurs when tetracycline antibiotics are administered during tooth development. The critical period for susceptibility to tetracycline-induced tooth discoloration is during tooth development, which occurs in utero and up to approximately 8 years of age. Tetracycline antibiotics, including tetracycline, doxycycline, and minocycline, can bind to calcium ions in developing teeth. This can lead to the formation of a stable, insoluble complex that is deposited in the dental enamel, leading to intrinsic tooth discolouration. Affected teeth may appear greyish or brownish in colour. The discoloration can range from mild to severe, depending on factors such as the dosage, duration of exposure and individual susceptibility. Tetracyclines are no longer antibiotics of choice in clinical dentistry due to their bacteriostatic activity and emergence of bacterial resistance.

Chlorhexidine continues to be one of the most popular antimicrobial agents in mouth-washes and is also used in toothpastes. Long-term use of chlorhexidine for over 4 weeks can lead to yellow-brown discolouration of teeth and should be avoided (see Chapter 11).

14.2.8 TASTE DISTURBANCES

Taste disturbances may be associated a wide variety of medications including:

- Antibiotics, e.g., azithromycin, aztreonam, clarithromycin, metronidazole
- Anticholinergics
- Antihypertensives, e.g., lisinopril, captopril
- Antithyroid drugs, e.g., thiouracil
- Baclofen
- Biguanide oral hypoglycaemics
- Cytotoxic drugs, e.g., cisplatin
- Penicillamine

Patients should be warned when prescribing antibiotics which may cause taste disturbances (e.g., metronidazole, azithromycin and clarithromycin etc.). If taste disturbances are suspected due to a systemic medication, advice from the prescribing physician may be sought to explore suitable alternatives. Taste disturbances may also be associated with xerostomia (see Chapter 13).

14.2.9 ORAL MELANIN PIGMENTATION

Melanin pigmentation of the oral mucosa may be enhanced by the following medications:

- Adrenocorticotropin hormone (ACTH)

- Heavy metals

- Oral contraceptives

- CCBs, e.g., amlodipine (see Figure 14.2)

- Phenothiazines, e.g., chlorpromazine thioridazine, trifluoperazine

- Zidovudine, (azidothymidine – AZT) an antiretroviral medication used in the prevention/ management of HIV/AIDS

14.2.10 MUCOSAL DISCOLOURATION

Superficial oral mucosal discolouration may manifest in a variety of colours as summarised as follows:

Blue/black discoloration may be caused by antimalarials (e.g., chloroquine), amiodarone, amodiaquine, bismuth, minocycline, sulfasalazine, lead, silver, tin and zinc. In addition, metal crowns and amalgam restorations (or amalgam fragments in oral soft tissues) may impart a dark discolouration to the oral mucosa.

Mucosal discoloration resulting from drug use may also manifest in the form of hairy tongue (Figure 14.3).

Apart from drugs, hairy tongue has many other causes such as tobacco use, poor oral hygiene, oxidising mouthwashes, etc., and may initially start as a yellowish discoloration of the tongue dorsum and may become progressively darker and change to a brown and black colour.

Green discoloration may be caused by copper.

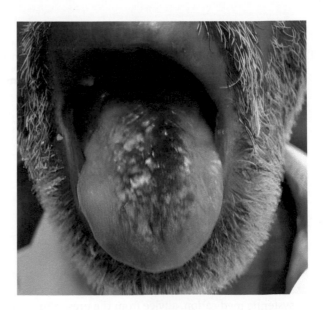

FIGURE 14.3 Hairy tongue in a patient on minocycline

14.2.11 DISCOLORATION OF SALIVA

Red or orange discolouration of saliva is reported with:

- Clofazimine
- Levodopa
- Rifabutin
- Rifampicin

14.2.12 SALIVARY GLAND SWELLING/PAIN

Salivary gland pain and swelling associated with drug use are uncommon but may be observed with:

- Buprenorphine
- H2 blockers (e.g., cimetidine)
- Insulin
- Methyldopa
- Naproxen
- Nifedipine
- Oxyphenbutazone
- Phenylbutazone
- Ranitidine

14.2.13 *HYPERSALIVATION* (PTYALISM)

Although uncommon, increased salivation may be associated with:

- Bethanechol
- Buprenorphine
- Digoxin
- Iodides
- Lamotrigine
- Mefenamic acid
- Modafinil
- Pilocarpine
- Venlafaxine

14.3 SUMMARY

Oral side effects that may be caused by a multitude of drugs, and it would be unrealistic to expect dental professionals to remember all the drugs that have these side effects. However, a summary of common and recognised oral effects of systemic medications have been discussed in the preceding sections. These side effects highlight the importance of accurately documenting a patient's drug history, and potential side effects of medications used by the patient must be ruled out when interpreting oro-facial signs and symptoms. Dentists must liaise with the patient's medical physician to discuss oral side effects of systemic medications and explore options for alternate drugs when appropriate.

14.4 SYSTEMIC MEDICATIONS ASSOCIATED WITH COMPLICATIONS FOLLOWING ORAL SURGICAL INTERVENTIONS

Some medications are associated with increased risk of complications following invasive dental and oral surgical procedures[6]. Examples include the following:

- *Bleeding tendency* in patients taking antiplatelets (e.g., aspirin, clopidogrel, dipyridamole, prasugrel and ticagrelor) and anticoagulants (e.g., warfarin, dabigatran, rivaroxaban, apixaban or heparin)[7]. Blood thinners are discussed separately in Chapter 15.

- *Medication-related osteonecrosis of jaws* (MRONJ) in patients taking bisphosphonates (e.g., alendronate, pamidronate and zoledronic acid), RANKL inhibitors (e.g., Prolia), and anti-angiogenic drugs (e.g., Bevacizumab and Sunitinib)[8]. MRONJ is discussed separately in Chapter 16.

ACKNOWLEDGEMENTS

Figure 14.1 provided by Dr Zubair Ahmed Khan, FMH College of Dentistry, Lahore Pakistan.
Figure 14.2 provided by Dr Gulraiz Zulfiqar, Jinnah Hospital, Lahore Pakistan.

RESOURCES

RESOURCES FOR DENTAL PROFESSIONALS

Food and Drug Authority. US drugs. https://www.fda.gov/drugs (accessed 25 February 2024).

RESOURCES FOR DENTAL PATIENTS

Mayo Clinic. Drugs. https://www.mayoclinic.org/drugs-supplements/drug-list (accessed 25 February 2024).

Patients should be encouraged to familiarise themselves with patient information leaflets (PILs) accompanying individual medications. Questions and concerns regarding the side effects and cautions may be discussed with the prescribing physician.

REFERENCES

1. SingleCare (2023). Prescription drug statistics 2023. https://www.singlecare.com/blog/news/prescription-drug-statistics (accessed 09 February 2024).

2. Statista (2000). England: prescription items dispensed 2006–2022. https://www.statista.com/statistics/418091/prescription-items-dispensed-in-england (accessed 10 February 2024).

3. Porter, S.R. and Scully, C. (2000). Adverse drug reactions in the mouth. *Clinics in Dermatology* 18: 525–532. https://doi.org/10.1016/S0738-081X(00)00143-7.

4. Teoh, L., Moses, G., and McCullough, M.J. (2019). A review and guide to drug-associated oral adverse effects—oral mucosal and lichenoid reactions. Part 2. *Journal of Oral Pathology and Medicine* 48: 637–646.

5. Abuhajar, E., Ali, K., Zulfiqar, G. et al. (2023). Management of chronic atrophic candidiasis (denture stomatitis)—a narrative review. *International Journal of Environmental Research and Public Health* 20: 3029. https://doi.org/10.3390/ijerph20043029.

6. Scottish Dental Clinical Effectiveness Programme (2021). Drug prescribing. www.sdcep.org.uk/published-guidance/drug-prescribing (accessed 10 February 2024).

7. Dézsi, C.A., Dézsi, B.B., and Dézsi, A.D. (2017). Management of dental patients receiving antiplatelet therapy or chronic oral anticoagulation: a review of the latest evidence. *European Journal of General Practice* 23: 197–202. https://doi.org/10.1080/13814788.2017.1350645.

8. Nicolatou-Galitis, O., Schiødt, M., Mendes, R.A. et al. (2019). Medication-related osteonecrosis of the jaw: definition and best practice for prevention, diagnosis, and treatment. *Oral Surgery, Oral Medicine, Oral Pathology and Oral Radiology* 127: 117–135. https://doi.org/10.1016/j.oooo.2018.09.008.

CHAPTER 15

Dental Management of Patients on Blood Thinners

Kamran Ali

Qatar University, QU Health, College of Dental Medicine, Doha, Qatar

15.1 INTRODUCTION

Blood thinners is a generic term which refers to antiplatelet and anticoagulant medications commonly used in the treatment and prophylaxis of cardiovascular disease to prevent thromboembolic events. Given that cardiovascular disease is common worldwide, dentists are likely to encounter patients who have been prescribed antiplatelet and anticoagulant medications. The most common indications for the use of these medications include the following:

- Ischaemic heart disease

- Prosthetic heart valves

- Cardiac arrhythmias

- Multiple deep vein thrombosis

- Multiple pulmonary emboli

- Some cases of ischaemic neurological disease, e.g., embolic strokes, transient ischaemic attacks

Routine minor oral surgical procedures in patients taking antiplatelet and anticoagulant medications carry a recognised risk of increased peri-operative and post-operative bleeding.[1, 2] Therefore, adequate patient preparation and precautions are warranted to avoid the risk of untoward bleeding following oral surgical interventions.

Contrary to the practice of interrupting antiplatelet and anticoagulant medications prior to the planned minor oral surgery procedures such as tooth extractions before the turn of the millennium, the current evidence suggest that interruption of these medications is associated with an increased risk of thromboembolic events and should be avoided.[3, 4] Bleeding complications from minor oral surgery, while undesirable, do not carry the same risks as thromboembolic complications, as the latter can be fatal. Patient preparation and appropriate precautions, including additional local haemostatic measures, can minimise the risk of bleeding in these patients allowing surgical interventions to be performed safely.[1, 5]

Whilst there is a wide range of antiplatelet and anticoagulant medications including those used in emergency management of acute cardiac events in hospital settings, dentists usually manage ambulatory patients in general practice settings. Therefore, this chapter will discuss the common oral antiplatelet and anticoagulant medications which are prescribed for long-term use. This is followed by guidance on performing minor oral surgery on patients taking these medications.

Clinical Dental Pharmacology, First Edition. Edited by Kamran Ali.
© 2024 John Wiley & Sons Ltd. Published 2024 by John Wiley & Sons Ltd.

Table 15.1 Common Oral Antiplatelet Agents

Drug	Mechanism of action	Standard dose	Half-life	Duration of effect (days)
Acetyl salicylic acid (Aspirin®)	Irreversible blockade of cycle-oxygenase-1 (COX1) and inhibition of thromboxane A2 (TXA2) synthesis	75 mg (EU) 81 mg (US)	20 min	7
Clopidogrel (Plavix®)	Irreversible inhibition of P2Y12 receptors on platelets	75 mg	~6 h	7
Prasugrel (Effient®)	Irreversible inhibition of P2Y12 receptors on platelets	10 mg	~7 h	7
Ticlopidine (Ticlid®)	Irreversible inhibition of P2Y12 receptors on platelets	250 mg twice daily	7–13 h	7
Ticagrelor (Brilique®)	Reversible inhibition of P2Y12 receptors on platelets	90 mg	6–13 h	1–2
Dipyridamole (Persantin®)	Reversible stimulation of cAMP synthesis	75–100 mg 4 times/day	8–15 h	1–2

15.2 ANTIPLATELET AGENTS

Platelets provide the initial haemostatic plug at the site of vascular injury. They are also involved in pathological processes and contribute to thromboembolic phenomenon leading to myocardial infarction and ischemic strokes. All antiplatelet medications affect haemostasis, but they do so by a variety of different mechanisms.

Platelet inhibition by antiplatelet agents may be reversible (e.g., aspirin, prasugrel, clopidogrel and ticlopidine) or reversible (e.g., dipyridamole, ticagrelor).

- *Irreversible inhibitors* bind covalently to the platelet receptors and deactivate it permanently, i.e., as long as it remains in circulation (even after the drug concentration has decreased).

- *Reversible inhibitors*, in contrast, bind to platelet receptors temporarily (binding and dissociation occur within minutes) and platelet function is restored as the blood levels of the drug decrease.

The mechanism of action, type of bond (irreversible/reversible) plasma half-life and duration of effect of common oral antiplatelet agents are summarised in Table 15.1.

15.3 ANTICOAGULANT AGENTS

Warfarin is the most common oral anticoagulant used by millions of people worldwide for over 50 years. In addition, other oral anticoagulants have been introduced subsequently including dabigatran apixaban and rivaroxaban. The mechanism of action and key features of these anticoagulants are summarised in Table 15.2.

INR provides a ratio of patient's prothrombin time (PT) compared to a control. INR in healthy individuals not on an anticoagulant range from 0.8 to 1.2. The therapeutic range of INR in patients placed on warfarin is usually from 2.0 to 4.0. INR is only suitable to monitor the activity of warfarin, while other anticoagulants require different tests for monitoring. Information on common drug interactions and contra-indications of anticoagulant agents is summarised in Table 15.3.

Table 15.2   Common Oral Anticoagulants

Drug	Mechanism of action	Reversal agent	Standard dose	Half-life (h)	Monitoring
Warfarin (Coumadin®)	Interferes with the activity of vitamin K-dependent clotting factors II, VII, IX and X; Protein C and S	Vitamin K	2–10 mg once daily	20–60	International normalised ration (INR)
Dabigatran Etexilate (Pradaxa®)	Inhibits free and clot-bound thrombin by binding to the active site of the thrombin molecule	Idarucizumab (Praxbind®)	150 mg tablet twice daily	12–17	Activated partial thromboplastin time (aPTT) and thrombin time (TT)
Rivaroxaban (Xarelto®)	Direct factor Xa inhibitor	Andexanet alfa (AndexXa®)	20 mg once daily	5–7	Activated partial thromboplastin time (aPTT) and anti-factor X-a assays
Apixaban (Eliquis®)	Reversible inhibitor of factor Xa	Andexanet alfa (AndexXa®)	5 mg tablet twice daily	12	Activated partial thromboplastin time (aPTT) and anti-factor X-a assays

Table 15.3   Oral Anticoagulants: Interactions and Contra-Indications

Drug	Increased anticoagulation	Decreased anticoagulation	Contraindications

Warfarin (Coumadin®)	Azole antifungals
	  Miconazole
	  Fluconazole
	  Ketoconazole
	Antibiotics
	  Erythromycin
	  Clarithromycin
	  Azithromycin
	  Metronidazole
	  Tetracycline
	  Cephalosporins
	NSAIDs
	  Aspirin,
	  Clopidogrel
	Alcohol
	Foods: Garlic
		Green leafy vegetables (high in vitamin K)	Other anticoagulants
			Aspirin
			Azole antifungals

Dabigatran Etexilate (Pradaxa®)	NSAIDs
	  Aspirin
	  Clopidogrel
	Ticagrelor
	  Clarithromycin
	Amiodarone
	Verapamil
	Quinidine
		Phenytoin
		Carbamazepine
		Rifampicin
			Other anticoagulants
			Azole antifungals
			HIV protease inhibitors

Rivaroxaban (Xarelto®)	NSAIDs
	  Aspirin
	  Clopidogrel
		Phenytoin
		Carbamazepine
		Rifampicin
			Other anticoagulants
			Azole antifungals
			HIV protease inhibitors

Apixaban (Eliquis®)	NSAIDs
	  Aspirin
	  Clopidogrel
		Phenytoin
		Carbamazepine
		Rifampicin
			Other anticoagulants
			Azole antifungals
			HIV protease inhibitors

15.4 DENTAL AND ORAL SURGICAL MANAGEMENT OF PATIENTS ON ANTIPLATELETS AND ANTICOAGULANTS

15.4.1 PRE-OPERATIVE ASSESSMENT AND PLANNING

- It is essential that dentists take a full medical history and identify patients on antiplatelet and anticoagulant medication(s).[6]

- Patients taking antiplatelet/anticoagulant medication with the following medical problems should not be treated in general dental practice settings and are best referred to local specialists for management in a hospital setting.
  - Liver impairment and/or alcoholism
  - Renal failure
  - Thrombocytopenia, haemophilia or any other systemic disorder of haemostasis
  - Patients taking a course of cytotoxic medication

- If there are any concerns regarding the patient's medical history including medication(s), consult with the patient's medical physician prior to carrying out any surgical procedure.

- Generally, antiplatelet/anticoagulant therapy should not be interrupted prior to minor oral surgical procedures due to the risk of acute cardiovascular events and the risk of bleeding can be minimised with additional haemostatic measures described later.

- Surgery should ideally be undertaken at the beginning of the day and the beginning of the week. This allows any re-bleeding to be dealt with during the working day or week.

ANTIPLATELET MEDICATION:

- If patients are taking aspirin alone or in combination with another antiplatelet medication (dual therapy), treat without interrupting the medication(s).

- Patients on triple antiplatelet therapy (rare) may require advice from their physician/specialist to stop one of the antiplatelet medications.

ANTICOAGULANT MEDICATION:

- Patients on warfarin need to get a pre-operative INR check ideally on the day of the surgical procedure but not earlier than 72 hours. In the United Kingdom, an INR less than 4.0 is considered the safe upper limit for minor oral surgical procedures like tooth extractions. However, in the United States, the safe upper limit of INR is 3.5.

- Anticoagulant activity of other drugs like dabigatran, rivaroxaban, or apixaban cannot be monitored with INR (see Table 15.2):
  - If the patient is on a twice daily dose of apixaban or dabigatran, the morning dose may be missed with the evening dose to be taken as usual.
  - If the patient is on a once daily dose of apixaban or dabigatran, the morning dose may be delayed for approximately 4 hours after haemostasis has been achieved.

15.4.2 PERI-OPERATIVE MANAGEMENT

- Following comprehensive pre-operative assessment and preparation described earlier, the following procedures can be carried out on patients taking antiplatelet/anticoagulant medications:
  - Simple extraction of up to three teeth,
  - Surgical placement of dental implants,

- Excision of a small soft tissue lump,
- Scaling and root planning of one quadrant,
- Pulp extirpation.

- All operative procedures should be performed with minimal trauma.

- If carrying out multiple extractions/implants, assess the severity of bleeding after each extraction/implant and only proceed to the next tooth, if bleeding is assessed to be manageable. Otherwise, consider staging the procedure at appropriate intervals. Similarly periodontal treatment should be done in stages.

- Local anaesthetic containing a vasoconstrictor (e.g., adrenaline) should be given by infiltration or intraligamentary injection, if practical. Inferior alveolar nerve blocks are best avoided due to the risk of hematoma formation in the pterygomandibular space.

- *Tooth extractions*: After tooth removal, take *additional measures to achieve haemostasis*:
  - The extraction socket should be packed gently with one of the local haemostatic agents:
    - Surgicel® (Regenerated oxidised cellulose)
    - Gelfoam® (Porcine gelatin sponge USP)
    - Hemocollagene® (Bovine collagen)
  Use of animal-based haemostatic agents should be discussed with the patients to ensure that it does not conflict with their cultural and religious values and principles:[7]
  - Each extraction socket should be sutured preferably using a horizontal mattress suture across the extraction socket(s).
  - Following closure, pressure should be applied to the socket(s) with a bite pack for 15 minutes.

- *Other procedures*:
  - The risk of bleeding in periodontal procedures can be minimised by infiltration of local anaesthetic with a vasoconstrictor. If there are concerns, post-operative bleeding can be addressed with the use of periodontal dressings such as Coe-pak™ or PerioCare®.
  - Pupal bleeding can also be controlled with the use of local anaesthetic with a vasoconstrictor either by application on cotton pellets or by infiltration.

- *Post-operative Care*
  - Haemostasis must be achieved prior to the patient leaving the surgery. It must be noted that in patients on anticoagulants, initial haemostasis may be achieved once a platelet plug has formed as platelet function in not impaired by anticoagulants, giving a false sense of reassurance. However, this may be followed by intractable bleeding if a fibrin clot fails to stabilise. Therefore, patients on anticoagulants need to be observed for longer, i.e., at least 30 minutes before discharging them home.
  - The patient should be given verbal and written post-operative instructions to reinforce precautions to prevent bleeding:
    - Avoid disturbing the wound with the tongue.
    - Avoid active spitting/rinsing of the mouth for the next 24 hours.
    - After 24 hours, gentle rinsing with warm saline may be done.
  - All patients should be provided out-of-hours contact details should the patient have any episodes of post-operative bleeding.
  - Beware of common drugs which may affect the activity of antiplatelet/anticoagulant drugs (Table 15.3) and take appropriate precautions. For example, paracetamol is recommended for post-operative analgesia. NSAIDs (e.g., aspirin and Ibuprofen) should be avoided.
  - If there are any concerns, a follow-up appointment should be made for the patient at the next available clinic.

15.5 SUMMARY

Dentists are likely to provide care to an increasing number of patients on blood thinners and should recognise the risks of bleeding following oral surgical interventions in these patients. Generally, antiplatelet and anticoagulant therapy should not be interrupted without medical advice. A vast majority of patients on antiplatelet and anticoagulant agents who require minor oral surgery, such as routine tooth extractions, can be treated safely in general dental practice settings. A comprehensive pre-operative assessment and an informed consent are essential prior to oral surgical interventions. Any concerns should be discussed with the patient's medical physician. Local measures are usually adequate to achieve haemostasis. Moreover, the patients should be provided detailed post-operative instructions to minimise the risk of bleeding. All patients should be provided contact details of local out of hours services should they experience uncontrolled bleeding.

RESOURCES

RESOURCES FOR DENTAL PROFESSIONALS

Scottish Dental Clinical Effectiveness Programme (SDCEP). Management of patients taking anticoagulants and antiplatelet drugs. www.sdcep.org.uk/published-guidance/anticoagulants-and-antiplatelets (accessed 25 February 2024).

RESOURCES FOR DENTAL PATIENTS

The American Academy of Oral Medicine (AAOMS). Blood thinners and dental care. https://www.aaom.com/index.php?option=com_content&view=article&id=126:blood-thinners-and-dental-care&catid=22:patient-condition-information&Itemid=120 (accessed 25 February 2024).

REFERENCES

1. Mauprivez, C., Khonsari, R.H., Razouk, O. et al. (2016). Management of dental extraction in patients undergoing anticoagulant oral direct treatment: a pilot study. *Oral Surgery, Oral Medicine, Oral Pathology, Oral Radiology* 122 (5): e146–e155.

2. Levi, M., Eerenberg, E., and Kamphuisen, P.W. (2011). Bleeding risk and reversal strategies for old and new anticoagulants and antiplatelet agents. *Journal of Thrombosis and Haemostasis* 9: 1705–1712.

3. Dudek, D., Marchionni, S., Gabriele, M. et al. (2016). Bleeding rate after tooth extraction in patients under oral anticoagulant therapy. *The Journal of Craniofacial Surgery* 27 (5): 1228–1233.

4. Sadhasivam, G., Bhushan, S., Chiang, K.C. et al. (2016). Clinical trial evaluating the risk of thromboembolic events during dental extractions. *Journal of Maxillofacial and Oral Surgery* 15 (4): 506–511.

5. Yoshikawa, H., Yoshida, M., Yasaka, M. et al. (2019). Safety of tooth extraction in patients receiving direct oral anticoagulant treatment versus warfarin: a prospective observation study. *International Journal of Oral and Maxillofacial Surgery* 48 (8): 1102–1108.

6. Scottish Dental Clinical (2022). Anticoagulants and antiplatelets. www.sdcep.org.uk/published-guidance/anticoagulants-and-antiplatelets (accessed 25 February 2024).

7. Ali, K., Gupta, P., Turay, E. et al. (2022). Dentistry in a multicultural society: the impact of animal-based products on person-centred care. *British Dental Journal* 232 (4): 269–272.

CHAPTER 16

Medication-Related Osteonecrosis of Jaws

Kamran Ali

Qatar University, QU Health, College of Dental Medicine, Doha, Qatar

16.1 INTRODUCTION

Medication-related osteonecrosis of jaw (MRONJ) was first identified in patients taking *bisphosphonates* in 2003 by oral and maxillofacial surgeons in the United States and was termed bisphosphonate-related osteonecrosis of jaw (BRONJ).[1,2] Subsequently, this complication was also identified with a wider range of medications including antiresorptive medications and anti-angiogenic agents; hence, the condition has been renamed as MRONJ.

Although MRONJ may develop spontaneously in patients taking these medications, a vast majority of cases develop as a complication following oral surgical interventions such as tooth extraction or bone surgery. The American Association of Oral and Maxillofacial Surgeons (AAOMS) uses the following criteria to diagnose MRONJ:[3]

1. Current or previous treatment with antiresorptive therapy alone or in combination with immune modulators or antiangiogenic medications.

2. Exposed bone or bone that can be probed through an intraoral or extraoral fistula(e) in the maxillofacial region that has persisted for more than 8 weeks.

3. No history of radiation therapy to the jaws or metastatic disease to the jaws

The relevant medications, their mechanism of action and indications are summarised in Table 16.1. It should be noted that the list is not exhaustive as new drugs are regularly emerging on the market. Dentists must always check the medications taken by the patients and should be clear on potential side effects of drugs, especially if drugs are likely to impact on provision of dental care.

16.2 RISK ASSESSMENT

The risk of MRONJ depends on both systemic and local factors as summarised in Table 16.2. A comprehensive approach is required for evaluation of the risk of MRONJ following dentoalveolar procedures. Cancer patients are at a higher risk of developing MRONJ compared to those with osteoporosis. The risk of developing MRONJ after tooth extraction in cancer patients has been reported to range from 1.6% to 14.8%.[4] On the other hand, tooth extractions in patients who take bisphosphonates for osteoporosis, the risk been reported to range from 0.02% to 0.05%.[5]

Clinical Dental Pharmacology, First Edition. Edited by Kamran Ali.
© 2024 John Wiley & Sons Ltd. Published 2024 by John Wiley & Sons Ltd.

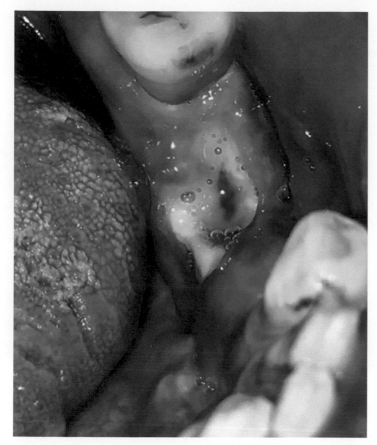

FIGURE 16.1   Ulceration and bone necrosis following extraction of lower left first molar. The patient was receiving intravenous zoledronic acid for bone pain associated with metastatic breast cancer

16.3 MANAGEMENT OF MRONJ

16.3.1 PRE-TREATMENT PREVENTION

Before commencement of antiresorptive or anti-angiogenic drug therapy, a comprehensive dental screening should be undertaken:

i. Educate patients on risks of MRONJ with antiresorptive and anti-angiogenic medications.

ii. Optimise oral health by achieving a meticulous oral hygiene, reduction in cariogenic diet, fluoride supplements, antimicrobial mouth rinses, smoking cessation, reduction in alcohol intake and regular dental check-ups.

iii. Identify and treat dental disease and remove existing or potential source(s) of infection, non-restorable teeth or those with poor prognosis may need to be extracted. This is particularly important for cancer patients who are at a higher risk of MRONJ following operative interventions once the patient has commenced therapy.

iv. If the patient requires extractions/osseous surgery, commencement of antiresorptive medication may need to be delayed until healing has been achieved. However, such decisions will need to be considered in the context of the patient's systemic condition and require a multidisciplinary approach.

Table 16.1 Medications Associated with Osteonecrosis of Jaws

Drug-group	Mechanism of action	Indications
I. Antiresorptive agents		
i. **Bisphosphonates**	Inhibit osteoclast differentiation and function and increase apoptosis.	• Osteoporosis • Osteopenia • Paget's disease, osteogenesis imperfecta

Oral
• Alendronic acid (*Fosamax*®
  Binosto® *Fosavance*®)
• Risedronate sodium
  (*Actonel*® *Actonel Combi*®)
• Etidronate (*Didronel*®)
 	
• Tiludronat (*Skelid*®)
	These actions lead to decrease bone resorption but also reduce remodelling capability of the bone. Oral surgical interventions carry a risk of MRONJ (Figure 16.1).	• Hypercalcaemia of malignancy,
		• Bone metastases
		• Lytic lesions of multiple myeloma

Intravenous
• Pamidronate disodium
  (*Aredia*®)
• Sodium Clodronate
  (*Bonefos*® *Clasteon*®
  Loron®)
• Ibandronic acid (*Bonviva*®
  Bondronat® *Quodixor*®)
• Zoledronic acid (*Zometa*®
  Aclasta®)		

ii. **Monoclonal antibodies** (Subcutaneous injection) • Denosumab (*Prolia*® *Xgeva*®)	Inhibits RANK-L (receptor activator of nuclear factor kappa-B ligand) responsible for formation/activation of osteoclasts and thereby reduces bone resorption.	• Osteoporosis • Bone metastases • Giant cell tumour of bone • Fibrous dysplasia
• Romosozumab (Evenity®)	Inhibits sclerostin, an endogenous cytokine which reduces bone formation and increases bone resorption. Romosozumab reverses these effects.	• Osteoporosis in post-menopausal women at elevated risk of bone fractures

II. Anti-angiogenic agents
• Bevacizumab (*Avastin*®)
  Intravenous injection
• Sunitinib (*Sutent*®)
  Oral administration
• Aflibercept (*Zaltrap*®)
  Trans conjunctival
	Interfere with the formation of new blood vessels and slow the growth of tumour cells.	• Bevacizumab and sunitinib are used for treatment of tumours involving the gastrointestinal, renal and neuroendocrine systems
		• Aflibercept is used for macular disease

Table 16.2   Risk Factors for MRONJ

Risk	Explanation
Systemic factors	
Antiresorptive medications	Intravenous route poses a higher risk than oral route.
	Longer duration of therapy increases the risk.
Co-morbidities	Cancer patients receiving antiresorptive medication have a recognised risk of developing MRONJ.
	Anaemia.
	Diabetes mellitus.
Concurrent medications	Corticosteroids and chemotherapy also increase the risk.
Smoking	Although conclusive evidence to implicate smoking as a risk factors for MRONJ is lacking, smoking cessation should be encouraged due to multiple health risks associated with smoking.
Local factors	
Dentoalveolar procedures	Risk mostly associated with tooth extractions and procedures involving alveolar bone.
	Risk with other interventions such as periodontal procedures, endodontics and implant placement not determined, but caution is advised especially in high-risk groups such as cancer patients.
Site	Risk higher in mandible than maxilla.
Presence of prosthesis	Risk higher in patients who wear dentures.
Periodontal disease	Insufficient evidence to implicate pre-existing periodontal disease to be regarded as a risk factor for MRONJ.

16.3.2 TREATMENT OF MRONJ

The management of MRONJ based on the clinical stages is summarised in Table 16.3. Dentists should refer established cases of MRONJ to oral and maxillofacial surgeons for management in specialist settings.

16.3.3 PROTOCOL FOR TOOTH EXTRACTIONS

Patients taking antiresorptive medications may require tooth extractions. Low-risk patients may be treated in general dental practice settings, high-risk patients including those with a history of cancer, are best managed in specialist settings.

A stepwise approach is described below:

- Establish that all other alternative treatment options have been considered.

- Evaluate the risk. Patients in the low-risk category may be treated by general dental practitioners. High-risk patients should be referred.

- Although there is no conclusive evidence to recommend drug holidays as a preventive measure to minimise the risk of MRONJ in patients requiring tooth extractions, this may be discussed with the relevant medical specialist responsible for prescribing antiresorptive medication.

- Obtain a valid and informed consent for extraction(s). Patients (or carer, as appropriate) should be advised regarding risk of developing MRONJ but reassure them the risk is small (generally less than 1% for low-risk category). Ensure the advice is understood by the patient and record appropriately in the consent and clinical notes.

Table 16.3 MRONJ Staging and Treatment

MRONJ staging	Treatment strategies
At risk category No apparent necrotic bone in patients who have been treated with either oral or IV bisphosphonates.	• No treatment indicated • Patient education
Stage 0 (Non-exposed bone) No clinical evidence of necrotic bone, but non-specific clinical findings (atypical odontalgia, dull ache involving the alveolar bone/sinus, neurosensory alterations, loosening of teeth, swelling), and radiographic changes (bone resorption not attributable to periodontal disease, reduced periodontal ligament space, sclerosis).	• Systemic management, including the use of pain medication
Stage 1 Exposed and necrotic bone or fistula extending to the bone, in patients who are asymptomatic and have no evidence of infection/inflammation Radiographic features of stage 0 may be present.	• Local care of exposed bone • Antimicrobial oral rinses • Removal of mobile/well-formed sequestrum
Stage 2 Exposed and necrotic bone or fistula extending to the bone and associated with infection as evidenced by pain and erythema in the region of the exposed bone with or without purulent drainage. Radiographic features of stage 0 may be present.	• Local care of exposed bone • Antimicrobial oral rinses, e.g., chlorhexidine • Removal of mobile/well-formed sequestrum • Systemic antibiotics • Pain control
Stage 3 Exposed and necrotic bone or fistula extending to the bone, with evidence of infection and one or more of the following: • Exposed and necrotic bone extending beyond the region of alveolar bone (i.e., inferior border and ramus in the mandible, maxillary sinus and zygoma). • Pathologic fracture. • Extra-oral fistula. • Oral antral/oral nasal communication. • Osteolysis extending to the inferior border of the mandible/sinus floor.	• Local care of exposed bone • Antimicrobial oral rinses • Removal of mobile/well-formed sequestrum • Systemic antibiotics (intravenous/oral) • Pain control • Consider surgical interventions, i.e., debridement/resection.

- Emphasise maintenance of excellent oral hygiene, smoking cessation and reduction in alcohol intake.

- The removal of a tooth should be performed with the least traumatic extraction technique and preferably one tooth at a time, or a sextant by – sextant approach.

- If obvious sharp socket wall margins or interradicular bone are observed following the procedure, these should be reduced selectively without lifting the periosteum from the bone.

- Antibiotics are not required in the low-risk group unless indicated for other reasons.

- The patient should be reviewed at appropriate intervals until the socket has healed completely.

- If the socket does not heal, or there are signs and symptoms of MRONJ, the patient should be referred appropriately.

ACKNOWLEDGEMENTS

Figure 16.1 provided by Dr Omer Janjua, Allied Hospital Faisalabad, Pakistan.

RESOURCES

RESOURCES FOR DENTAL PROFESSIONALS

American Association of Oral and Maxillofacial Surgeons (AAMOS). Medication-related osteonecrosis of the Jaw – 2022 update. https://www.joms.org/article/S0278-2391(22)00148-3/pdf (accessed 21 March 2024).

Scottish Dental Clinical Effectiveness Programme (SDCP). Oral health management of patients at risk of medication-related osteonecrosis of the Jaw. https://www.sdcep.org.uk/published-guidance/medication-related-osteonecrosis-of-the-jaw/ (accessed 25 February 2024).

RESOURCES FOR DENTAL PATIENTS

Mayo Clinic. Osteoporosis treatment: medications can help. https://www.mayoclinic.org/diseases-conditions/osteoporosis/in-depth/osteoporosis-treatment/art-20046869#:˜:text=Bisphosphona-tes%20and%20denosumab%20can%20also,or%20other%20invasive%20dental%20work (accessed 25 February 2024).

REFERENCES

1. Ruggiero, S.L., Mehrotra, B., Rosenberg, T.J., and Engroff, S.L. (2004). Osteonecrosis of the jaws associated with the use of bisphosphonates: a review of 63 cases. *Journal of Oral and Maxillofacial Surgery* 62 (5): 527–534.

2. Dannemann, C., Grätz, K.W., Riener, M.O., and Zwahlen, R.A. (2007). Jaw osteonecrosis related to bisphosphonate therapy. A severe secondary disorder. *Bone* 40 (4): 828–834.

3. Ruggiero, S.L., Dodson, T.B., Aghaloo, T. et al. (2022). American Association of Oral and Maxillofacial Surgeons' position paper on medication-related osteonecrosis of the jaws—2022 update. *Journal of Oral and Maxillofacial Surgery* 80: 920–943.

4. Scoletta, M., Arata, V., Arduino, P.G. et al. (2013). Tooth extractions in intravenous bisphosphonate-treated patients: a refined protocol. *Journal of Oral and Maxillofacial Surgery* 71 (6): 994–999.

5. Hallmer, F., Andersson, G., Götrick, B. et al. (2018). Prevalence, initiating factor, and treatment outcome of medication-related osteonecrosis of the jaw—a 4-year prospective study. *Oral Radiology* 126 (6): 477–485.

Medical Emergencies

Management of Medical Emergencies

CHAPTER 17

Kamran Ali

Qatar University, QU Health, College of Dental Medicine, Doha, Qatar

17.1 INTRODUCTION

The occurrence of medical emergencies in dental practice is recognised worldwide. Dentistry involves treating human beings with dental problems and is associated with potential risks. All efforts must be directed at prevention of medical emergencies in the first place. It is equally important that the dental staff is trained and prepared to deal with medical emergencies. The latter demands the availability of emergency equipment and drugs onsite and prompt access to medical help.

With improved healthcare facilities at the present time, dentists (and other clinical dental professionals) are much more likely to encounter patients with recognised medical problems. In a way this has made life easier for dentists as most patients with systemic diseases are already diagnosed and would often narrate their medical problems sometimes even without being prompted. Nevertheless, a large section of the population still remains undiagnosed in early stages of certain diseases, such as hypertension and diabetes mellitus, and the dentists must play their role as oral physicians in early recognition and appropriate referral to the medical colleagues.

It is mandatory to obtain a thorough medical history and carry out a physical examination at the first visit and update medical records regularly. If recording medical history is delegated to another colleague, the clinician treating the patient must confirm the medical history with the patient before commencing treatment. Ideally, patients should have their vital signs recorded at the first visit and periodically as dictated by changes in their medical status. Although dentists do not record vital signs routinely, it is a highly useful approach and can help to identify potential medical problems at an early stage and seek medical advice.[1] It is crucial that if required, the dentists liaise with the medical colleagues to seek advice regarding the medical status of their patients.

In the developed countries, access to emergency medical help is readily available and a large number of patients with potentially fatal medical emergencies are able to survive with prompt medical support. In locations where access emergency services are unavailable, emergency medical help may be organised by liaising with nearby hospitals or medical clinics. However, in such cases the dental practitioner must ascertain the nature and quality of the services available in the medical facility including the best possible manner to access these, i.e., transport of patient or otherwise. In locations where access to emergency medical help is not readily available, it may be very difficult to locate and contact medical services during an emergency if this has not been already organised.

Clinical Dental Pharmacology, First Edition. Edited by Kamran Ali.
© 2024 John Wiley & Sons Ltd. Published 2024 by John Wiley & Sons Ltd.

17.1.1 GENERAL GUIDELINES ON MANAGEMENT OF MEDICAL EMERGENCIES IN DENTAL PRACTICE

1. Prevention is the cornerstone of management.

2. Always review medical history before commencing dental treatment.

3. Consider seeking medical advice when indicated by medical history of patients.

4. Be prepared to deal with emergencies.

5. Ensure dentists and ancillary staff are trained for emergency procedures.

6. Clear and maintain airway.

7. Perform basic life support (BLS) and use an external automated defibrillator.

8. Training should be repeated at least annually. Training in medical emergencies is a statutory requirement for dental professionals globally and must be undertaken with a certified provider.

9. Ensure all drugs and equipment are stored appropriately and organised for easy access and use.

10. Never work alone.

11. Ensure there is easy access to emergency ambulance service for medical help.

12. If a patient collapses at any stage, check for signs of life (breathing and circulation) and if there are no signs of life, provide Cardiopulmonary resuscitation (CPR).

13. Keep abreast of changes in practice by continuing education and training.

14. Record contemporaneous clinical notes to document the occurrence and management of medical emergencies including help from emergency services.

15. Undertake regular clinical audits to review and enhance preparedness for the management of medical emergencies in clinical dental settings.

17.1.2 EMERGENCY EQUIPMENT FOR DENTAL SURGERY

GENERAL:

- Telephone with emergency number at hand.
- Watch or clock with second hand.
- Automated external defibrillator (AED).
- Portable suction with appropriate attachments, e.g., the Yankauer suction tip.
- Blood pressure recording device.
- Pulse oximeter.
- Glucometer.

OXYGEN ADMINISTRATION:

- Portable oxygen cylinder (D size) with pressure reduction valve and flowmeter.
- Oxygen face mask with reservoir and tubing.
- Pocket mask with oxygen port.

- Self-inflating bag and mask apparatus with oxygen reservoir and tubing (1 L size bag).

- Adult and child face masks for attaching to self-inflating bag.

- Oropharyngeal airways: Guedel airways sizes 1–4.

INHALATIONAL DRUG ADMINISTRATION:

- Spacer device for inhaled bronchodilators.

DRUG ADMINISTRATION:

- Single use plastic syringes (5 and 10 mL) and needles (18 and 21 gauge).

17.1.3 EMERGENCY DRUGS

PARENTERAL:

Sympathomimetic: Adrenaline injection 1.0 mg/mL (1:1000 solution).

Antihypoglycaemic: Glucagon injection 1 mg vials for i.m administration.

Anticonvulsant: Midazolam 10 mg in 2 mL vials.

ORAL:

Antihypoglycemic: Oral glucose solution, powder, gel (Hypostop).

Antiplatelet: Aspirin dispersible tablets (300 mg).

Anticonvulsant: Midazolam buccal tablets (10 mg).

Vasodilator: Glyceryl trinitrate (GTN) spray (400 μg/dose).

INHALATIONAL

Oxygen

Bronchodilator: Salbutamol (Ventolin) inhaler (100 μg/actuation).

In most countries, dentists are not required to administer drugs by intravenous route. This is because intravenous route carries additional risks and dentists may not have adequate skills and/or confidence to administer drugs intravenously in emergency situations. Medical emergencies in dental practice can be managed safely with administration of appropriate drugs using the oral, inhalation and intramuscular route. However, skills in intravenous drug administration may offer some advantages in the management of medical emergencies and may be used by dentists with appropriate training depending on local legislation and guidelines.

17.2 PATIENT ASSESSMENT

A thorough clinical assessment is crucial to manage medical emergencies, and the A–E approach is considered to be appropriate for assessing patients experiencing medical emergencies in dental practice settings.[1]

- **A**irway

- **B**reathing

- **C**irculation

- **D**isability

- **E**xposure

ABCDE assessment is summarised in Table 17.1

Table 17.1 ABCDE Assessment of Patients Experiencing Medical Emergencies

Component	Assessment	Recognised abnormalities
Airway	Check airway patency and identify any obstruction • Open the airway using the head tilt, chin lift manoeuvre or jaw thrust (suspected cervical spine injury) • Remove any visible and accessible foreign bodies using finger swipe and use of high-volume suction to clear blood, vomitus, etc.	• Airway may be obstructed by foreign bodies, blood or vomitus • Deterioration in conscious level may allow the tongue to fall back and obstruct the airway • Airway obstruction may also result from dislodgement of dental restorations, materials or tooth fragments down the aerodigestive tract. • Airway obstruction causes paradoxical (see-saw) chest and abdominal movements and use of accessory muscles of respiration
Breathing	Check rate, depth, symmetry and pattern of breathing (Normal breathing rate 12–20 breaths/minute in adults and 20–30 in children) Note any abnormal breath sounds	• Tachypnoea: anxiety, asthma, COPD, IHD, diabetic ketoacidosis • Bradyopnoea: OSA, drug overdose, head injury • Wheeze – high-pitched whistling sound due to narrowing of airways, usually on expiration (asthma, bronchitis) • Stridor – noisy breathing usually on inspiration (laryngeal obstruction/stenosis) • Gurgling – bubbling or rattling noise during breathing due to fluid in upper airways (aspiration, pleural inflammation) • Snoring – vibrating sound due to narrowing of oropharyngeal airways (tongue fall) as observed during sleep
Circulation	• Check skin colour and temperature • Check capillary refill time (CRT) by pressing on the patient's fingertip for 5 seconds to make the tissue blanch; then release the pressure and note the time for the blood flow to be restored – indicated by the return of normal skin colour – usually <2 seconds. • Check rate, depth, regularity of peripheral pulse (normal heart rate 60–100 beats/minute in adults)	• CRT >2 seconds indicates poor peripheral perfusion • Tachycardia: anxiety, anaemia, fever, hypovolaemia, hypoxia, asthma, COPD, hyperthyroidism, drugs, caffeine, alcohol • Bradycardia: athletes, myocardial ischaemia, hypothyroidism
Disability	• Check level of consciousness using AVPU **A**lert; responds to **V**erbal prompt; responds to **P**ain, or **U**nresponsive • Measure blood glucose; levels below 70 mg/dL or 3.9 mmol/L indicate hypoglycaemia	• Deterioration of consciousness may be related to vasovagal fainting (transient), hypoglycaemia • Weakness of face, arms and a slurred speech may indicate CVA • Loss of consciousness with loss of breathing/pulse may indicate a cardiac arrest
Exposure	Look for any swelling, skin rashes or bleeding	• Skin rashes, erythema and urticaria may indicate an allergic reaction or anaphylaxis

17.3 VASOVAGAL SYNCOPE

Vasovagal fainting or syncope is the most common cause of sudden loss of consciousness and up to 2% patients faint before or during dental treatment.

17.3.1 PREDISPOSING FACTORS

- Physical/emotional stress (injections)
- Fear (injections)
- Anxiety
- Pain (injections)
- Fatigue
- Starvation
- Mental illness
- High temperature and relative humidity

Contrary to the popular belief, hypoglycemia is usually not involved but must be ruled out in all suspected cases.

17.3.2 PATHOPHYSIOLOGY

Stress and anxiety associated with dental treatment (e.g., fear of dental injections) may lead to *vasovagal fainting* or *syncope*. It is a biphasic response characterised initially by an increased sympathetic tone followed by the activation of the parasympathetic system (Figure 17.1).

Mass discharge of impulses mediated by the hypothalamus stimulate the release of adrenaline from the adrenal glands into blood circulation resulting in vasodilation in skeletal muscles (β_2 receptors) leading to peripheral pooling of blood and reduced venous return. This is followed by vasoconstriction in the skin (α_1 receptors) leading to pallor and ashen grey appearance of the face, increased rate and force of heart contraction (β_1 receptors).

The vigorous contractions of 'empty' ventricles stimulate C fibres in the left ventricle, increasing the vagal tone which overrides the sympathetic activity causing a reduction in venous return and consequent cerebral ischemia. The *fainting reflex* helps to divert blood to the brain by causing the patient to fall to the ground, which allows restoration of cerebral circulation and recovery. The vasovagal attack is transient and benign and rarely last for more than a few minutes. However, it could prove to be fatal if a patient is maintained in an upright position in a dental chair due to permanent cerebral damage secondary to ischemia.

17.3.3 SYMPTOMS

- Premonitory dizziness
- Weakness
- Nausea

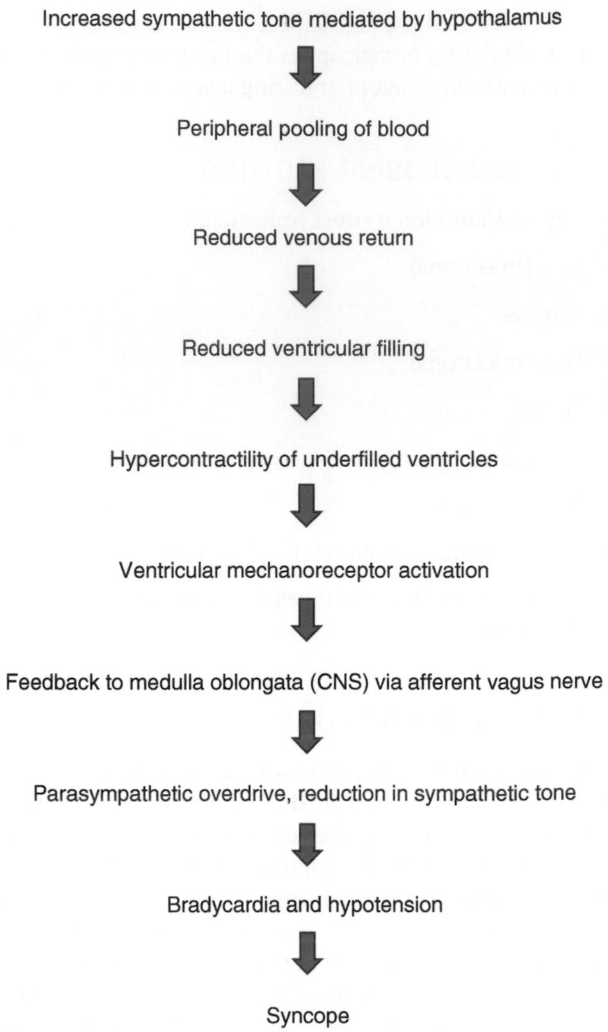

Increased sympathetic tone mediated by hypothalamus

Peripheral pooling of blood

Reduced venous return

Reduced ventricular filling

Hypercontractility of underfilled ventricles

Ventricular mechanoreceptor activation

Feedback to medulla oblongata (CNS) via afferent vagus nerve

Parasympathetic overdrive, reduction in sympathetic tone

Bradycardia and hypotension

Syncope

FIGURE 17.1   Pathophysiology of vasovagal syncope

17.3.4 SIGNS

- Skin pallor (Ashen colour)
- Sweating
- Confusion
- Vomiting
- Pulse initially rapid and full (increased sympathetic activity) but becomes slow and weak (increased parasympathetic tone).
- Fall in blood pressure
- Loss of consciousness (within 2–3 minutes)
- Seizures (if unconsciousness is prolonged)

17.3.5 MANAGEMENT

Most episodes of vasovagal syncope can be prevented by calm reassurance and effective communication with the patient prior to dental treatment:

- Carefully explain the nature of the procedure.

- Administer all local anaesthetic injections with the patient in supine position (as explained in Chapter 3).

- Keep the patient under direct observation and maintain verbal contact with the patient throughout the dental procedure to monitor their well-being.

- Stop the treatment immediately if the patient becomes stressed or unwell at any stage during the treatment.

Management of an episode of syncope is summarised in Box 17.1.

BOX 17.1   **MANAGEMENT OF VASOVAGAL SYNCOPE**

1. Terminate all dental treatment.
2. Place the patient in supine posture as soon as possible with the legs raised to improve the venous return and restore the cerebral circulation (Figure 17.2).
3. Loosen tight clothing, especially around the neck.
4. Administer oxygen (15 L/minutes).

Patient recovers   *No recovery*

Reassurance   Check pulse and respiration
Continue treatment, or   Clear airway
reschedule the appointment   Consider other causes of syncope
                                                          Assess need for CPR
                                                          Call for help

---

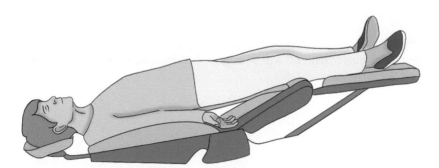

FIGURE 17.2   Chair positioning to restore cerebral circulation in syncope

17.3.6 DIFFERENTIAL DIAGNOSIS

Other conditions associated with syncope include

1. Hypotension (postural)

2. Hypoglycaemia

3. Myocardial Infarction

4. Cardiac arrest

5. Bradycardia or heart block

6. Stroke

7. Epilepsy

8. Adrenocortical insufficiency

9. Drug reactions

   The probable cause of collapse in each case may be indicated by the patient's medical history:

- *Postural (orthostatic) hypotension* is characterised by sudden fall in blood pressure when standing up from a sitting or lying position. It may be observed in patients taking antihypertensive medications (e.g., ACE inhibitors, angiotensin antagonists), use of recreational drugs, pregnancy, old age, Addison's disease and diabetic patients with autonomic neurotherapy. Patients receiving dental treatment in a supine position are particularly susceptible to postural hypotension when standing up which may lead to syncope. Patients receiving dental treatment should be returned to sitting position slowly and must take their time when rising from the chair.

- *Hypoglycaemia* may cause collapse in a diabetic patient especially around mealtimes (discussed later).

- *Myocardial infarction* might be responsible for collapse in a patient with a history of ischaemic heart disease and may progress to a cardiac arrest, especially if complicated by ventricular fibrillation (VF) (discussed later).

- Adrenocortical insufficiency may lead to collapse in patients with primary Addison's disease or those taking steroid therapy.

   In most cases, prevention/management of syncope is fairly straightforward. However, a dentist may end up in a stressful situation if the medical history of the patient has not been recorded appropriately prior to commencing treatment, especially if there is no one accompanying the patient.

17.4 ACUTE CHEST PAIN

Acute chest pain might be precipitated in patients with a previous history of ischaemic heart disease (angina pectoris or myocardial infarction).

17.4.1 SYMPTOMS

- Chest pain
- Palpitations
- Breathlessness
- Sweating

17.4.2 SIGNS

- Changes in heart rate (bradycardia or tachycardia)

- Irregular pulse

- Dyspnoea

- Low blood pressure

- Increased capillary refill time

- Changes in conscious level

The symptoms of myocardial infarction are more marked compared to transient pain associated with angina pectoris. Chest pain associated with myocardial infarction is more severe and progressive and may radiate to the shoulder, arm (usually left side), neck, lower jaw and through to the back. In addition, the patient may appear pale, clammy and experience nausea and vomiting.

17.4.3 MANAGEMENT

The management of acute chest pain secondary to ischaemic heart disease is summarised in Box 17.2.

BOX 17.2	MANAGEMENT OF ACUTE CHEST PAIN

1. Stop all dental procedures.
2. Let the patient decide the most comfortable position. If the patient is breathless, they may prefer to sit upright. However, if the patient feels faint, it may be better to lay them flat.
3. Reassure the patient to reduce anxiety.
4. Give patient GTN spray (400 µg) sublingually and wait 2–3 minutes.
5. Administer oxygen (15 L per minute) especially if there is evidence of cyanosis or deterioration in conscious level.
6. Additional doses of GTN spray may be administered at 3–5-minute intervals if required.

Pain relieved

Consider rescheduling the appointment
Advise consultation with the medical physician

Pain not relieved
(Pain worsens/patient becomes unstable)

Call for medical help
Administer aspirin tablet 300mg orally crushed or chewed
If the patient collapses at any stage, check for signs of life (breathing, and circulation) and if there are no signs of life, provide CPR.

17.4.4 DIFFERENTIAL DIAGNOSIS

In addition to ischemic heart disease, acute chest pain may be associated with the other conditions as shown in Table 17.2.

Table 17.2 Differential Diagnosis of Acute Chest Pain

Cardiovascular system
Pericarditis
Aortic aneurysm

Respiratory system
Pulmonary embolism
Pleuritis
Tracheobronchitis
Mediastinitis
Pneumothorax

Gastrointestinal system
Dyspepsia
Reflex oesophagitis
Gastric ulcers

Musculoskeletal system
Intercostal muscle spasm
Osteochondritis

Psychogenic

17.5 CARDIAC ARREST

Cardiac arrest is defined as a sudden and complete loss of cardiac function. It is characterised by:

1. Loss of consciousness

2. Absence of pulse

3. Immediate cessation of respiration

Cardiac arrest is always fatal unless treated promptly.

17.5.1 CAUSES

- VF characterised by rapid, ineffective uncoordinated movement of ventricles. VF can be caused my myocardial infarction or electrocution.

- Ventricular asystole (VA) characterised by cessation of electrical activity of the ventricles. It can result from massive ventricular damage after myocardial infarction.

- Pulseless electric activity (PEA) characterised by lack of effective cardiac output despite normal or near-normal electrical activity. PEA can develop as a complication of pericardial tamponade, cardiac rupture, massive pulmonary embolism (PE), anaesthetic overdose, tension pneumothorax, electrolyte imbalance and hypothermia.

17.5.2 MANAGEMENT

Prompt management is required to prevent irreversible brain damage (up to 3 minutes). CPR protocol in dental settings involves BLS. All dentists must be trained to carry out BLS manoeuvres including the use of an AED as a mandatory requirement. Nowadays, in most countries, even the general public and schoolchildren are also trained in BLS measures. Dentists who provide sedation

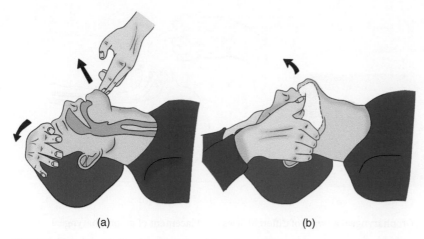

(a)   (b)

FIGURE 17.3   Head tilt, chin lift (a) and jaw thrust (b) manoeuvres to open the airway

services are expected to receive additional training on intermediate life support (ILS). Advanced life support (ALS) is provided by specialised medical teams experienced in providing CPR.

Basic Life Support

CPR using chest compressions and AED is used universally by first aiders to 'buy time' in resuscitation of people who experience a cardiac arrest. Effective CPR can help to sustain a person until more expert medical treatment is available. The sequence of BLS in adults is summarised in Figure 17.3.

1. *Ensure it is safe to approach the victim.*

2. *Check responsiveness* (shake the shoulders and ask loudly 'Are you all right?'). If there is no response, ask for nearby help.

3. *Turn the patient onto their back and then open the airway:*
    a. *Head tilt and chin lift:* Place one hand on the forehead of the collapsed individual and gently tilt the head back while the fingertips of the other hand are placed under the chin and the chin is lifted to open the airway (Figure 17.3a).
    b. *Jaw thrust:* Place two fingers of each hand close to the angle of mandible and push the jaw forward. It is used if a cervical spine injury is suspected. (Figure 17.3b).
    - Clear airway of mucus, blood, vomitus and debris.
    - Quickly use two fingers to gently sweep it away from the mouth.
    - Alternatively, use a high-volume suction.
    - If large amounts of debris/vomitus are present and a high-volume suction is not available, the casualty may be turned into the recovery position (explained later) to help clear debris and drain vomit.
    - Dentures are best left in position as these help to provide a seal when trying to ventilate a casualty and are only removed if they are ill fitting.
    - If the victim's tongue is falling back and obstructing the airway, select an oropharyngeal airway of an appropriate size (Figure 17.4a). The correct size may be determined by estimating the distance from the angle of the mouth to the angle of the mandible and place it in situ to keep the airway patient (Figure 17.4b).

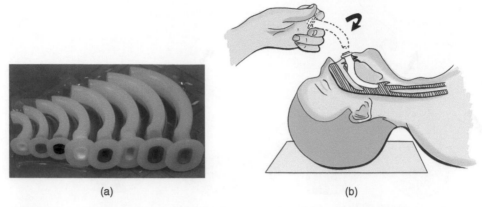

(a) (b)

FIGURE 17.4 Oropharyngeal airways of different sizes (a). Placement of an oropharyngeal airway (b)

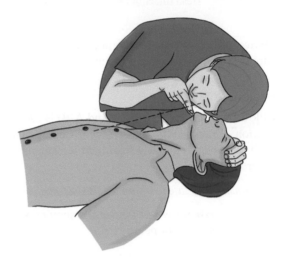

FIGURE 17.5 Checking for breathing

4. *Keeping the airway open, assess breathing for no more than 10 seconds* (Figure 17.5).

Look for chest movement.
Listen for breath sounds the patient's mouth.
Feel for expired air on your cheek.

Cardiac arrest should be suspected if the person is unresponsive breathing is absent or abnormal, i.e., slow laboured breathing (agonal gasping). Send a helper to call an ambulance and bring an AED.

A brief period of seizure-like activity may also be observed immediately following a cardiac arrest. Once seizures stop, reassess responsiveness and breathing.

5. *Start CPR with chest compressions as soon as possible.*

Ideally the victim should be placed on a firm flat surface, e.g., floor in a clear and accessible position. If the victim is too heavy to be lifted out of the dental chair, resuscitation may be carried out in the dental chair in supine position (chair fully reclined).

Place the heel of one hand in the centre of the victim's chest (lower half of the sternum) as shown in Figure 17.6.

Place the heel of your other hand on top of the first hand and interlock the fingers of your hands (Figure 17.7).

Avoid direct pressure on ribs/lower end of the sternum or the upper abdomen.

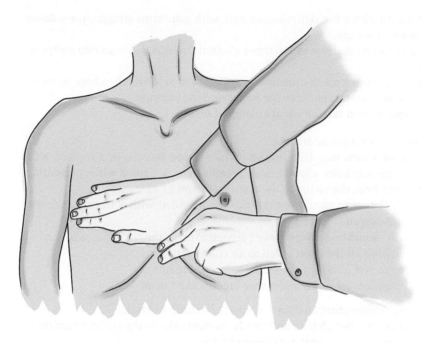

FIGURE 17.6 Identifying the correct spot for chest compressions

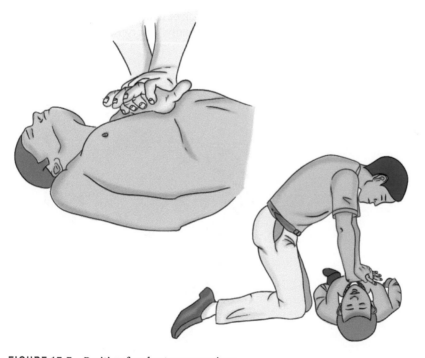

FIGURE 17.7 Position for chest compressions

Position yourself vertically above the victim's chest and, with your arms straight, press down on the chest to a depth of 5–6 cm.

Provide 30 chest compressions at a rate of 100 times a minute (a little less than two compressions per second).

After each compression, release all the pressure on the chest to allow the chest to recoil completely without losing contact between the hands and the sternum.

Compression and release should take an equal amount of time.

6. *Combine chest compression with rescue breaths.*

   Thirty chest compressions may be followed by two rescue breaths in a ratio of 30:2. A pocket mask with a one-way valve allows rescue breaths to be delivered while preventing backflow of air/secretions from the victim to the rescuer (Figure 17.8).

   Alternatively, ventilation in dental settings may be provided with a bag valve device along with supplemental oxygen (Figure 17.9).

   Each rescue breath should be delivered over 1 second to make the chest rise as in normal breathing and then watching for the chest to fall as air comes out.

   Repeat once more to give a total of two effective rescue breaths.

   Continue with chest compressions and rescue breaths at a rate of 30:2.

7. *Use an AED as soon as possible (ideally within 3 minutes of a cardiac arrest).*
   a. As soon as the AED arrives, switch it on and attach the electrodes to the victim's bare chest as depicted on the chest pads/defibrillator (Figure 17.10).
   b. Follow the instructions of the AED (interrupt chest compressions, stand clear of the victim, allow the AED to assess the heart rhythm and deliver a shock if instructed).
   c. Resume CPR immediately after the shock is delivered (or otherwise) until instructed by the AED to stop CPR (usually 2 minutes) for another check of heart rhythm.
   d. Stop to re-check the victim only if they start breathing normally; otherwise, do not interrupt resuscitation.

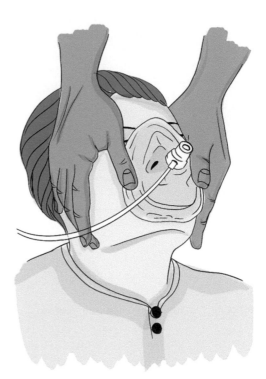

FIGURE 17.8 Oxygen mask

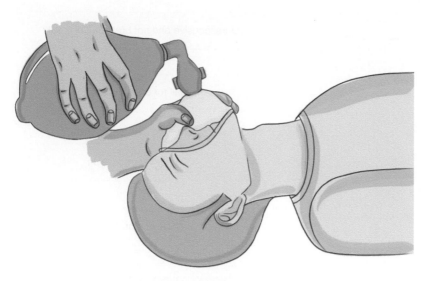

FIGURE 17.9 Bag-valve mask ventilation

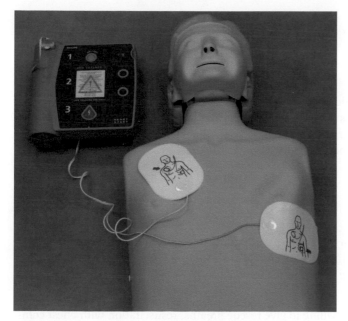

FIGURE 17.10 Automated external defibrillator

8. If there is more than one rescuer present, another should take over CPR about every 2 minutes to prevent fatigue. Ensure there is a minimum delay during the changeover of rescuers.

9. *Continue resuscitation until:*

   Help arrives and the ambulance staff take over,
   The victim starts breathing normally, or
   The rescuer(s) become exhausted.

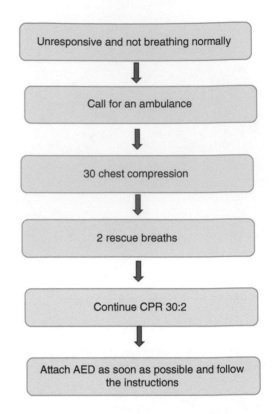

FIGURE 17.11 Adult Basic Life Support Algorithm

The resuscitation council UK does not require the rescuers providing BLS to check the pulse (Figure 17.11).[2] Although there is less stress on a pulse check in the BLS algorithm by the American Heart Association (AHA), rescuers are still expected to check the pulse for 5–10 seconds. As mentioned before, dental professionals should always follow local guidelines when managing medical emergencies.

Explanatory Notes

- *Agonal gasps*:

    Agonal gasps are present in up to 40% of cardiac arrest victims and may occur in the first few minutes after sudden cardiac arrest. CPR should not be delayed if the victim is unconscious (unresponsive) and not breathing normally. It should be emphasised that agonal gasps.

- *Chest-compression-only CPR*:

    If a rescuer is unable or unwilling to give rescue breaths, resuscitation with chest compressions only may be carried out as it be as effective as combined ventilation and compression in the first few minutes after a non-asphyxial arrest.

- *Bag-mask ventilation*:

    Considerable practice and skill are required to use a bag and mask for ventilation and ideally requires two rescuers. If appropriately trained, a lone rescuer can open the airway with a jaw thrust whilst simultaneously holding the mask to the victim's face.

- *Automated External Defibrillator*:

    An AED is a portable electronic device designed to treat sudden cardiac arrest. It delivers an electrical shock to the heart to restore its normal rhythm. AEDs are user-friendly devices which are designed to be used individuals with basic training in emergency situations including lay people. Public awareness, training and accessibility of AEDs are important factors in improving survival rates for sudden cardiac arrest.

When turned on, an AED provides clear, step-by-step voice instructions and/or visual prompts through a screen or indicator lights. The adhesive electrode pads are placed on the victim's bare chest following the images on the pads or the defibrillator. These pads contain sensors that analyse the heart's electrical activity to determine if the victim's heart rhythm is a shockable rhythm, i.e., can respond positively to defibrillation (such as ventricular fibrillation or ventricular tachycardia).

- *Shock advised*: If a shockable rhythm is detected, it will prompt the user to stand clear and press a button to deliver an electrical shock to the heart. This shock aims to stop the chaotic rhythm and allow the heart's natural pacemaker to re-establish a normal rhythm.
- *No shock advised*: If a shock is not needed, it will advise the rescuer to continue CPR until emergency medical help arrives.

Paediatric BLS

The following key points should be noted when providing BLS for infants and children.[3]

- Provide five rescue breaths before commencing chest compressions

- Use a ratio of 15 chest compressions (100–120/minute) and two rescue breaths

- The depth of chest compressions in infants is 4 cm and 5 cm in children

- Use two fingers for chest compression in infants and one to two hands in children

- If the rescuer is not trained/confident in paediatric BLS, adults BLS protocol may be used with appropriate modifications to the depth and force of chest compressions.

Recovery Position

Following successful resuscitation, if at any time the casualty vomits, they will need to be put into the recovery position so that their airway can be cleared until medical help arrives. Figure 17.12 depicts the steps in placing a victim in recovery position.

17.6 CHOKING AND ASPIRATION

The close proximity of the oral cavity to the airway poses a high risk of aspiration and/or airway obstruction during dental treatment. Additionally, the use of local anaesthetics may diminish sensations in the oropharynx and impair the cough reflex. Aspiration and/or airway obstruction may result from blood, tooth fragments during extractions, implants, dental materials (e.g., impression material), instruments (e.g., endodontic files) etc. Appropriate precautions must be observed at all times to protect the airway. Depending on the dental procedure these may include use of rubber dam, high volume suction, tongue depressor and more importantly vigilance on behalf of the operator and the dental assistant.

17.6.1 SYMPTOMS

- Cough or splutter

- Difficulty in breathing

- Clutching of the neck

- Expression of anxiety and fear

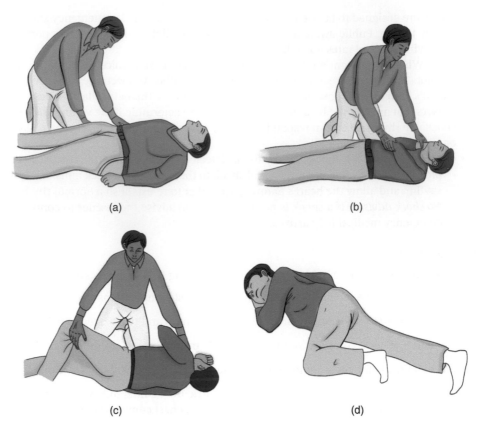

(a)

(b)

(c)

(d)

FIGURE 17.12   Steps for placing a patient into a recovery position. (a) Place the nearside arm with palm upwards underneath the near side; (b) draw the other arm across placing the back of the palm against the cheek and temple; (c) draw the far knee upward keeping the other leg straight and gently roll the body towards yourself with the hand supporting the head; and (d) extend the head in the sniffing the morning air position to allow good air entry

17.6.2 SIGNS

- Abnormal breath sounds, e.g., wheezing (aspiration) or stridor (upper airway obstruction)
- Paradoxical chest/abdominal movements
- Severe cases
  - Unable to cough
  - Cyanosis
  - Altered conscious level
  - Cardiorespiratory arrest

A foreign body is more likely to lodge in the right bronchus as it is more vertical and in line with the trachea.

17.6.3 MANAGEMENT

The management of choking is dependent on the severity of obstruction as summarised in Figure 17.13 If the source of obstruction is visible and easily accessible it may be removed carefully with a finger swipe and/or use of high-volume suction.

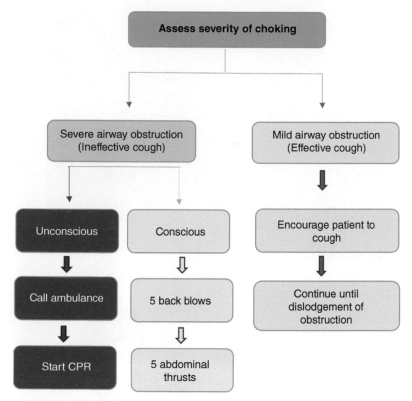

FIGURE 17.13   Algorithm for management of choking in adults

Mild Airway Obstruction

Encourage the patient to continue coughing until the obstruction relieved. If the patient deteriorates, manage as for severe obstruction.

Severe Airway Obstruction

Patient is conscious
Give up to five back blows.

- Stand to the side and slightly behind the victim

- Support the chest with one hand and lean the victim well forwards so that when the obstructing object is dislodged it comes out of the mouth rather than goes further down the airway (Figure 17.14).

- Give up to five sharp blows between the shoulder blades with the heel of your other hand and observe for dislodgement/relief of obstruction after each back blow.

Give up to five abdominal thrusts.

- Stand behind the victim and put both arms round the upper part of his abdomen (Figure 17.15).

- Lean the victim forwards.

- Clench your fist and place it between the umbilicus (navel) and the bottom end of the sternum (breastbone).

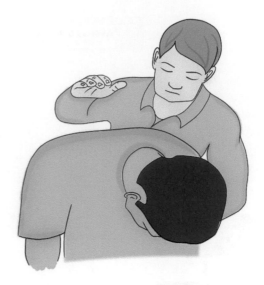

FIGURE 17.14 Back blows to clear respiratory obstruction in adults

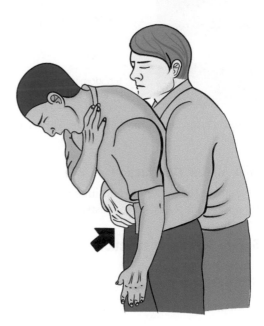

FIGURE 17.15 Abdominal thrusts to clear respiratory obstruction in adults

- Grasp this hand with your other hand and pull sharply inwards and upwards.

- Repeat up to five times, checking for dislodgement/relief of obstruction after each abdominal thrust.

    If the obstruction is still not relieved, continue alternating five back blows with five abdominal thrusts.

    Patient is unconscious

- Support the victim carefully to the ground.

- Immediately call an ambulance.

- Start CPR.

Following successful treatment for choking, foreign material may nevertheless remain in the upper or lower respiratory tract and cause complications later. Patients who have aspirated foreign bodies (e.g., a tooth or a fragment of dental material/instrument) or show symptoms (persistent cough, difficulty in swallowing) should be referred urgently to a local hospital for medical assessment, chest radiograph and removal of foreign bodies using bronchoscopy if indicated. Moreover, abdominal thrusts can potentially cause serious injuries to the internal organs and patients receiving abdominal thrusts should be examined by a medical professional to rule out such injuries.

There are some differences in the management of choking in infants and children which are summarised below:

- *Back blows in an infant:*
  - A rescuer should support the infant in a head-downwards, prone position. The infant's head should be supported by placing the non-dominant hand on the lower jaw
  - Deliver up to five sharp back blows with the heel of one hand in the middle of the back between the shoulder blades, checking between each blow if the obstruction is relieved (Figure 17.16).

- Back blows in a child over 1 year:
  - Position the child with the head down and deliver five back blows as for an infant

If obstruction is not relieved with back blows, give chest thrusts to infants or abdominal thrusts to children.

- *Chest thrusts in an Infant*
  - Position the infant into a head-downwards supine position (Figure 17.17).
  - Deliver up to five chest thrusts (lower sternum, one finger's breadth above the xiphisternum), checking between each thrust, if the obstruction is relieved.

- *Abdominal thrusts for children over 1 year:*
  - Stand behind the child and place a clenched fist between the umbilicus and xiphisternum. Grasp your fist with your other hand and pull sharply inwards and upwards up to five times, checking between each thrust, if the obstruction is relieved.
  - If the object has not been expelled and the victim is still conscious, continue the sequence of back blows and chest (for infant) or abdominal (for children) thrusts.
  - If the child/infant with airway obstruction is, or becomes, unconscious, call for emergency help and start paediatric BLS.
  - As for adults, children and infants who have the obstruction removed successfully, should be assessed at the hospital by medical professionals.

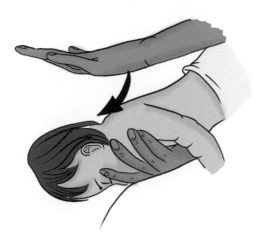

FIGURE 17.16 Back blows to clear respiratory obstruction in infants and children

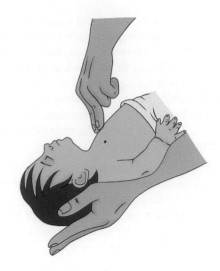

FIGURE 17.17 Chest thrusts to clear respiratory obstruction in infants

17.7 ACUTE ASTHMA

Asthma is observed in children as well as adults. Asthmatic patients have very sensitive airways, and when they are exposed to certain triggers, their airways narrow due to broncho-constriction making it difficult for them to breathe. An episode of acute asthma may well be precipitated during dental treatment.

17.7.1 PRECIPITATING FACTORS

- Anxiety
- Exercise
- Emotion
- Infection especially viral infections of upper respiratory tract
- Sudden exposure to an allergen
- Drugs, e.g., aspirin and beta-blockers

17.7.2 SYMPTOMS

- Anxiety
- Breathlessness
- Difficulty in completing a sentence in a single breath
- Chest tightness/pain
- Frequent cough

17.7.3 SIGNS

- Wheezing
- Tachycardia (>110/minute)

- Sweating
- Intercostal retraction
- Life threatening asthma may be present with the following signs
  - Bradycardia (<50/minute)
  - Chest may be silent in severe asthma due to insufficient air flow
  - Slow breathing (<8/minute)
- Rapid shallow breathing (>25/minute)
- Peripheral cyanosis (lips/face)
- Confusion and deterioration of conscious level
- Collapse – leading to eventual respiratory arrest

17.7.4 MANAGEMENT

The management of acute asthma is summarised in Box 17.3.

BOX 17.3   **MANAGEMENT OF ACUTE ASTHMA**

- Reassurance to calm the patients.
- Position the patient upright; do not lay the patient flat as it makes breathing more difficult.
- Administer salbutamol inhaler (100 µg/actuation) preferably using a large spacer device as it can improve deposition of a drug to lower airways significantly. This may be repeated as necessary and up to 10 activations may be given.
- Oxygen administration (15 L/minute).

Patient shows improvement

Continue treatment or
Reschedule the appointment

No improvement

Call for medical help

Continue administration of oxygen, and salbutamol inhaler every 10 minutes until help arrives.

If bronchospasm is accompanied by signs of anaphylaxis, consider administration of adrenaline 1:1000 by intramuscular injection (see management of anaphylaxis)

If the patient becomes unresponsive, check for 'signs of life' (breathing and circulation) and if absent, start CPR.

17.8 HYPERVENTILATION

Hyperventilation is characterised by quick, shallow breaths from the top of the chest which reduce the level of carbon dioxide in the blood. This reduced level of carbon dioxide may lead to respiratory alkalosis causing the arteries to constrict and reduce the flow of blood throughout the body. Hyperventilation usually affects individuals with anxiety, fear or emotional outbursts.

17.8.1 PRESENTATION

- Anxiety
- Rapid breathing
- Rapid pulse
- Pressure, tightness or pain across the chest
- Dry mouth
- Prolonged hyperventilation may lead to:
  - Blurred vision
  - Tingling in fingers and toes
  - Fainting

17.8.2 MANAGEMENT

Reassurance of the patient and a calm approach often leads to quick relief.

- Reassurance
- Remove the cause of anxiety if possible
- Guide the patient through controlled breathing exercises, (slow, deep breaths through the nose, hold for few seconds, and exhale slowly through the mouth).
- Do not use a paper or plastic bag for rebreathing. This may lead to suffocation especially in children

17.9 ANAPHYLAXIS

Anaphylaxis is a rapidly developing, generalised hypersensitivity reaction with life-threatening effects on the airways, breathing and circulation along with skin and mucosal involvement. Anaphylaxis may develop within minutes following exposure to an allergen and requires immediate treatment.

17.9.1 PATHOGENESIS

Anaphylaxis is a rapidly developing immunologic reaction (Type I) occurring within minutes after the combination of an antigen with IgE antibodies bound to mast cells or basophils in individuals previously sensitised to the antigen. It results in the degranulation of mast cells and release of histamine and other inflammatory mediators leading to serious clinical manifestations related airway involvement, breathing difficulties, and circulatory problems.

Typically, anaphylaxis occurs on the second or third exposure to the drug, even in very small amounts. Although anaphylaxis can be triggered by a variety of allergens, the most recognised causes in dentistry include administration of drugs, e.g., penicillin, and exposure to latex, chlorhexidine, eugenol and benzocaine topical anaesthetic gel.

Fortunately, allergy to amide local anaesthetic is relatively rare. Again, a thorough medical history to identify any allergies to drugs or medicine and avoidance of suspected agents is essential to avoid allergic reactions.

17.9.2 SYMPTOMS

- Facial flushing

- Itching

- Numbness

- Cold extremities

- Breathlessness

- Nausea, vomiting, abdominal pain and diarrhoea

- A sense of impending doom

17.9.3 SIGNS

- Facial swelling

- Rashes with urticaria, erythema,

- Cold clammy skin

- Thready pulse

- Laryngeal oedema with wheezing, stridor and hoarseness of voice

- Bronchospasm

- Hypotension due to widespread vasodilation, may lead to collapse

- Cardiac arrest may result from hypovolemia or respiratory arrest

17.9.4 MANAGEMENT

The management of anaphylaxis is summarised the Box 17.4.

BOX 17.4	MANAGEMENT OF ANAPHYLAXIS

Use ABCDE approach to confirm diagnosis

Call for help

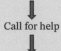

Lay patient flat with legs raised (unless there is breathing impairment/vomiting)

↓

Administer adrenaline (1:1000) by IM injection (vastus lateralis muscle on the anterolateral aspect of middle third of thigh)

Adult and child >12 years	500 μg (0.5 mL)
Child 6–12 years	300 μg (0.3 mL)
Child <6 years	150 μg

Alternatively, use a preloaded EpiPen injection (300 μg adrenaline) (0.15 mL).

- Adrenaline injection may be repeated after 5 minutes if no improvement is observed.
- Maintain airway with 100% oxygen (15 L/minute).
- If the patient is experiencing severe breathing difficulties, salbutamol inhaler (100 μg) may be administered using a spacer device as for acute asthma.
- If the patient becomes unresponsive, check for 'signs of life' (breathing and circulation) and if absent, start CPR.

17.10 HYPOGLYCAEMIA

Hypoglycaemic collapse is most commonly seen in diabetic patients. Hypoglycaemia may impair brain function rapidly as brain is solely dependent on glucose for energy. The possible causes of hypoglycaemia in diabetes mellitus include:

- Missed, delayed or inadequate meal

- Insulin overdose/inappropriate regime

- Unusual exercise

- Malabsorption

- Alcohol

17.10.1 PRESENTATION

The presentation of hypoglycaemia is summarised in Table 17.3. Features of hyperglycaemia are also included for comparison.

A prompt and accurate diagnosis of hypoglycaemia can be made with a glucometer and thus guide the clinician regarding the most appropriate management strategy. Although the precise value of blood glucose at which patients develop features of hypoglycaemia may vary amongst individuals, a blood glucose level <3.0 mmol/L is diagnostic of hypoglycaemia.

Table 17.3   A Comparison of Clinical Presentation of Hypoglycaemia and Hyperglycaemia

Assessment	Hypoglycaemia	Hyperglycaemia
Causes	Missed meals, insulin overdose, unusual exercise, malabsorption	Missed, insufficient insulin, excessive glucose intake
Onset	Rapid onset	Slow onset
Presentation	Irritability and aggression	Drowsiness and disorientation
	Moist sweaty skin	Dry skin, dry mouth
	Pulse full and rapid	Pulse weak and rapid
	Dysarthria	Acetone breath; ketonuria
	Normal or high blood pressure	Hypotension
	Headache; neurological fits	Abdominal pain
	Normal or shallow breathing	Hyperventilation
	Loss of consciousness (rapid)	Loss of consciousness (slow)
Glucose measurements	Blood sugar low (usually <3.0 mmol/L (54 mg/dL))	Blood sugar high (usually >20 mmol/L (360 mg/dL))

17.10.2 MANAGEMENT

The management of hypoglycaemia is summarised in Box 17.5.

BOX 17.5   **MANAGEMENT OF HYPOGLYCAEMIA**

1. Terminate all dental treatment
2. Lay patient flat
3. Confirm diagnosis (blood glucose measurement with a glucometer)

Patient Conscious	*Impaired Consciousness*
(Co-operative with an intact gag reflex)	(Uncooperative, impaired gag reflex)

Patient Conscious

Give oral glucose such as,[a]
- Sugar (sucrose) 25 g
- Milk with added sugar
- Glucose tablets/or gel

Repeat after 10–15 minutes.

Check blood glucose again in 10 minutes and ensure it is >5mmol/L.

Impaired Consciousness

Give glucagon IM[b]
Adults 1 mg
Child >8 year or 25 kg 1 mg
Child <8 years or < 25 kg 0.5 mg

If the patient recovers and is able to swallow, provide oral glucose.[a]

Check blood glucose again in 10 minutes and ensure it is >5mmol/L.

Seek medical help if no recovery.

If the patient is unconscious, check for signs of life and provide CPR if signs of life are absent.

ᵃOral glucose

Examples of oral glucose include 5 glucose tablets, 200 mL of fruit juice (with normal sugar content, not sugar-free or reduced-sugar), 3–4 teaspoonfuls of sugar added to a cup of water and 2 tubes of glucose 40% gel (such as Glucogel®, or Dextrogel®).

ᵇGlucagon injection

- Inject the liquid from the syringe through the rubber stopper of the vial, shake the vial without removing the needle until a clear mixture is visible.

- Push the plunger full and before withdrawing all the solution back into the syringe.

- Remove any air bubbles by pointing the needle upwards, tapping the syringe with your fingers and pushing the plunger until the correct dose is ready to be administered.

- Administer the injection intramuscularly in either the shoulder (deltoid) or in the buttocks (gluteus maximus).

It is important to reiterate that following glucagon administration, the recovery may be brief and there is a risk that the patient may experience hypoglycaemia again. If the patient is able to swallow, oral glucose must be administered because if the patient loses consciousness again, a repeat glucagon injection may not be effective due to insufficient glycogen stores in the patient's body.

If the patient recovers, the appointment may be rescheduled and the patient sent home preferably with an accompanying adult family member or a friend. The patient's medical physician must be informed and the patient advised to avoid driving for the rest of the day.

17.10.3 DIFFERENTIAL DIAGNOSIS

Hypoglycaemia may be associated with a variety of other conditions as shown in Table 17.4.

Table 17.4 Other Causes of Hypoglycaemia

Pancreatic disease
  Insulinoma
  Islet hyperplasia
  Pancreatitis

Autoimmune hypoglycaemia
  Autoimmune insulin syndrome
  Anti-insulin receptor antibodies

Essential reactive hypoglycaemia
  Post-gastrectomy
  GIT mobility disorders

Endocrine disease
  Pituitary insufficiency
  Adrenocortical insufficiency
  Hypothyroidism

Miscellaneous
  Hepatocellular disease,
  Advanced renal failure
  Prolonged starvation, e.g., anorexia nervosa
  Alcohol
  Excessive exercise

17.11 ADRENAL INSUFFICIENCY

Adrenal insufficiency may lead to collapse of a patient during or prior to dental treatment. The possible causes include:

- Primary Addison's disease
- Systemic corticosteroid therapy (most common)
- Post-adrenalectomy
- Hypopituitarism

17.11.1 PREDISPOSING FACTORS

- Stress
- Trauma
- Anaesthesia
- Surgery
- Infection

17.11.2 SYMPTOMS

- Profound weakness
- Lack of well-being
- Nausea
- Abdominal pain
- Dizziness

17.11.3 SIGNS

- Pallor
- Irregular, weak and rapid pulse
- Rapidly progressive hypotension
- Vomiting
- Altered consciousness

17.11.4 MANAGEMENT

Prevention

Most patients on low doses of systemic steroids can undergo routine dental treatment in outpatient settings without the need for a steroid cover. However, patients who are susceptible to adrenal insufficiency during dental treatment need to be evaluated for the need for a steroid cover to prevent this complication. Steroid cover is required for patients with primary Addison's disease, patients on high dose of steroids, following adrenalectomy, and if treatment is provided under general anaesthesia.

Treatment

The treatment of acute adrenal insufficiency requires replacement therapy with parenteral fluids, glucose and steroids based on measurement plasma electrolytes and glucose. However, dental surgeries are usually not equipped to provide this treatment. Therefore, patients with adrenal insufficiency in dental settings are usually managed with the following:

1. Use ABCDE approach to assess the patient and confirm diagnosis.

2. Summon medical help.

3. Lay patient flat with legs raised (unless vomiting).

4. Give oxygen at 15 L/minute.

5. If the patient becomes unresponsive, check for signs of life and provide CPR if signs of life are absent.

17.12 EPILEPTIC SEIZURES

Epilepsy encompasses a group of disorders in which there are recurrent episodes of seizures due to altered cerebral function associated with paroxysmal excessive and hypersynchronous discharge of cerebral neurons. The cause of epilepsy may not be evident in the majority of the cases but may include head injuries, stroke, brain tumours, infections such as meningitis or injury during childbirth.

An epileptic seizure may be precipitated during a dental appointment in those with generalised (tonic-clonic seizures) and sometimes partial complex seizures.

17.12.1 PRECIPITATING FACTORS

- Starvation (hypoglycaemia)
- Inappropriate anti-epileptic medication
- Acute hypoxia
- Alcohol
- Photosensitivity

17.12.2 SIGNS AND SYMPTOMS

- A seizure may be preceded by a warning sensation or aura involving visual, auditory, olfactory, gustatory or somatosensory sensations.
- The subject may utter a cry and fall if not in the dental chair.
- Loss of consciousness with generalised rigidity and cyanosis (tonic phase). Trauma to the tongue may occur due to inadvertent biting.
- Convulsions follow with jerking movements (clonic phase) for up to several minutes.
- Frothing from the mouth and urinary incontinence may be observed.
- Consciousness is usually regained after few minutes, but the patient may remain drowsy and confused for several hours.

17.12.3 MANAGEMENT

The aim of management during an epileptic seizure is to prevent the patients injuring themselves and to maintain a clear airway, most fits terminate spontaneously. The management of an epileptic seizure is summarised in Box 17.6.

BOX 17.6   **MANAGEMENT OF EPILEPTIC FIT**

---

1. Clear the area around the patient to prevent injury during convulsions
    o Do not attempt to restrain the patient
    o Do not attempt to insert anything in the mouth or between the teeth
2. Oxygen administration at 15 L per minute
3. Check blood glucose level and administer glucose gel or glucagon IM if blood glucose is <3.0 mmol/L

Convulsions subside	Convulsions continue (≥5 minutes) or recur

Wait for full recovery
Reschedule the appointment
Send home accompanied
Consider hospital referral:
First episode of seizure
Additional concerns.

Call for help.
Administer buccal midazolam.

> Adults/children>10 years 10 mg
> Children 5–10 years 7.5 mg
> Children 1–5 years 5 mg

If the patient becomes unresponsive, check for 'signs of life' (breathing and circulation) and if absent, start CPR.

17.12.4 DIFFERENTIAL DIAGNOSIS

Seizures may be observed in the following conditions due to cerebral damage:

- Untreated hypoglycaemia
- Poorly managed vasovagal syncope
- Cardiorespiratory arrest

17.13 CEREBROVASCULAR ACCIDENT

Cerebrovascular accident (CVA) results from damage to brain either due to cerebral haemorrhage or infarction (ischemia) and is one of the leading causes of death worldwide. Although CVA is a rare occurrence during dental treatment, it requires emergency help for life-saving treatment and prevention of long-term disability.

17.13.1 CAUSES

- Intracranial haemorrhage secondary to hypertension (most important)
- Cerebral embolism

- Cortico-vertebral insufficiency
- Subarachnoid haemorrhage

17.13.2 SYMPTOMS

- Light-headedness
- Headache
- Slurring of speech

17.13.3 SIGNS

- Weakness of face
- Weakness of limbs, e.g., unable to raise the arms
- Loss of consciousness
- Dilated, unequal pupils (larger on the affected side)
- Urinary/faecal incontinence

17.13.4 MANAGEMENT

1. Call for help
2. Maintain a clear airway
3. Administer oxygen
4. If the patient becomes unresponsive, check for 'signs of life' (breathing and circulation) and if absent, start CPR. In the UK, public education campaigns use the acronym FAST to recognise people with suspected stroke and seek prompt medical help.

    'Lives can be saved by learning to think and act FAST'

Face – has the face fallen on one side?

Arms – can they raise both arms and keep them there?

Speech – is the speech slurred?

Time – call for emergency helpline (999 in the United Kingdom).

ACKNOWLEDGEMENTS

Figures 17.2, 17.3, 17.4, 17.5, 17.6, 17.7, 17.8, 17.9, 17.12, 17.14, 17.15, 17.16 and 17.17 produced by Miss Shahd Ali R N Al-Najdi, Qatar University, Doha Qatar

RESOURCES

RESOURCES FOR DENTAL PROFESSIONALS

- Resuscitation Council UK. Professional resources. www.resus.org.uk/professional-resources (accessed 26 February 2024).

- American Heart Association. CPR and first aid – emergency cardiovascular care. https://cpr.heart.org/en/ (accessed 26 February 2024).

- Addison's Self-Help Group. www.addisonsdisease.org.uk/addisons-disease-advice-for-dentists (accessed 26 February 2024).

REFERENCES

1. Resuscitation Council UK (2021). ABCDE approach. www.resus.org.uk/library/abcde-approach (accessed 26 February 2024).

2. Resuscitation Council UK (2021). Adult basic life support. www.resus.org.uk/library/2021-resuscitation-guidelines/adult-basic-life-support-guidelines (accessed 26 February 2024).

3. Resuscitation Council UK (2021). Paediatric basic life support. www.resus.org.uk/library/2021-resuscitation-guidelines/paediatric-basic-life-support-guidelines (accessed 26 February 2024).

Prescription Writing

Dentists frequently prescribe drugs to patients and must ensure that the drug prescriptions are issued after careful consideration of patient's medical history and recognition of issues which may affect drug compliance. Meticulous attention to detail is crucial to ensure patient safety and effective treatment. Inappropriate/unsafe prescriptions may be flagged up by pharmacists dispensing the drugs causing unnecessary delays and inconvenience to the patients. In some less developed countries, professional oversight by pharmacists may not be always available, and in such circumstances the dentists have an even greater responsibility to ensure that their drug prescriptions are safe and appropriate.

- Evaluate patient's medical history and concurrent medications to ensure the prescribed drugs are safe, there is no known risk of allergy or drug interactions with patient's existing medication(s) such as oral anticoagulants (see Chapter 15). Seek medical advice if unsure.

- Special considerations and precautions are required for pregnant and breastfeeding women; children, and elderly; and for patients with systemic disease especially hepato-renal disorders.

- Discuss the common and any serious side effects of drugs to be prescribed with the patient or their carer prior to prescribing.

- Consider relevant national professional guidelines and statutory regulations to ensure only drugs permissible for prescription by dentists are prescribed.

- Use appropriate prescription forms if required by professional regulations.

- Over-the-counter medications, e.g., common analgesics, may be cheaper for patients. Only prescribe when necessary.

  The following information should be included on the drug prescriptions:

- *Patient Information*:
  Include the patient's full name, date of birth and any relevant identification numbers or codes (e.g., medical record number).

- *Date*:
  Write the date on which the prescription is issued to facilitate documentation, tracking (if required) and audit of drug prescriptions.

- *Prescriber Information*:
  Include the full name, professional title, contact information, and, if applicable, professional license number of the prescriber.

Clinical Dental Pharmacology, First Edition. Edited by Kamran Ali.
© 2024 John Wiley & Sons Ltd. Published 2024 by John Wiley & Sons Ltd.

- *Details of Drug(s) Prescribed*:
    - i. Name of the drug(s) – use generic names whenever possible.
    - ii. The exact dose.
    - iii. Strength (concentration).
    - iv. Route of drug administration (usually oral or topical is used).
    - v. Formulation (capsule, tablet or suspension).
    - vi. Frequency and timing.
    - vii. Drugs to be taken as required must have a minimal dose interval.
    - viii. Duration of treatment (days/weeks).
    - ix. Mention the diagnosis/clinical indication for which the medication is prescribed (optional).
    - x. Total quantity of the medication(s) to be dispensed.
    - xi. Include important instructions, precautions or and warnings for use.
    - xii. Encourage patients to read patient information leaflets accompanying the prescribed medication(s).

- *Signature*:
    Sign the prescription (on paper or electronically) with your full name and professional title. This is a legal requirement in many countries.
    Additionally, handwritten prescriptions must be legible and written and signed using a pen with indelible ink.

APPENDIX B
Drug Prescriptions in Elderly Patients

Elderly patients may have additional challenges due to physical and mental changes that accompany old age and may be taking multiple prescribed medications, increasing the risk of unwanted/serious drug interactions. The following points may be considered in elderly patients:

- Tailor medication choices to the individual patient, considering their specific health conditions, preferences and goals.

- Evaluate ability to swallow.

- Prescribe from a limited range.

- Be familiar with the side effects of prescribed medications on the elderly.

- Dosages may be lower than for younger patients.

- Be vigilant for signs of adverse drug reactions, especially in the first few weeks of starting a new medication.

- Review repeat prescriptions regularly.

- Prescribe simple treatment regimens, e.g., once or twice daily whenever possible.

- Write full instructions on the prescription so that the container can be labelled properly.

- Avoid child-proof containers for medicines as elderly patients may find it difficult to manage them.

Clinical Dental Pharmacology, First Edition. Edited by Kamran Ali.
© 2024 John Wiley & Sons Ltd. Published 2024 by John Wiley & Sons Ltd.

Drug Prescriptions in Children

- Children's doses are lower than adults and may need to be determined by their body weight and surface area.

- Liquid preparations may be easier to swallow than capsules or tablets. Alternatively, choose chewable tablets, if available.

- Use sugar-free formulations if possible.

- Avoid prescribing aspirin in children due to the risk of Reye's syndrome.

- Do not add medicines to infant's feed as some medicines may interact with milk or other liquids and interfere with the child's ability to finish the meal.

- Provide clear and detailed instructions to parents or caregivers on how to administer the medication. Include information on dosing, frequency and any special instructions.

- Discuss the importance of medication adherence with parents or caregivers and schedule regular follow-up appointments to monitor progress.

- Advise parents and caregivers to keep all medicines out of the reach of children.

Clinical Dental Pharmacology, First Edition. Edited by Kamran Ali.
© 2024 John Wiley & Sons Ltd. Published 2024 by John Wiley & Sons Ltd.

Drug Prescriptions During Pregnancy

Prescribing drugs during pregnancy requires careful consideration to balance the potential benefits to the mother against the potential risks to the developing foetus. No drug is completely free of side effects and drugs should be prescribed only when absolutely necessary. The main considerations are as follows:

- Evaluate the potential benefits of treatment for the mother against the potential risks to the developing foetus.

- Consider the timing of exposure. Early pregnancy (first trimester) is the most critical period for foetal development, so minimise drug exposure during this time.

- Be aware of drugs known to be teratogenic (causing birth defects) and avoid them. Provide alternative treatments if available.

- Ensure the mother's health is optimised by consulting with the patient's medical physician if there are any concerns.

- Consider the likelihood of the drug crossing the placental barrier and its potential effects on foetal development.

- If a medication is deemed necessary, aim for the lowest effective dose to minimise potential risks (Table D.1).

- Consult with relevant specialists, such as patient's gynaecology specialist or teratology information services, for complex cases or when uncertainty exists.

- Clearly document discussions with the patient regarding the potential risks and benefits of any prescribed medication during pregnancy.

Clinical Dental Pharmacology, First Edition. Edited by Kamran Ali.
© 2024 John Wiley & Sons Ltd. Published 2024 by John Wiley & Sons Ltd.

Table D.1 Drug Prescription During Pregnancy

Category	Avoid	Suitable alternatives
Analgesics	Non-steroidal anti-inflammatory drugs, e.g., aspirin (risk of Reye's syndrome), ibuprofen, Opioids, e.g., codeine	Paracetamol
Antibiotics	Tetracyclines (risk of tooth discolouration) Metronidazole (first trimester)	Penicillins, e.g., amoxicillin Cephalosporins Macrolides, e.g., azithromycin Clindamycin
Local anaesthetics	Articaine	Lidocaine

Drug Prescriptions to Breastfeeding Mothers

As with pregnancy, prescribing drugs during breastfeeding requires careful consideration to balance the potential benefits to the mother against the potential risks to the breastfeeding infant. No drug is completely free of side effects and drugs should be prescribed only when absolutely necessary. The main considerations are as follows:

- Be aware of the potential for drugs to transfer into breast milk, consider non-pharmacological alternatives or medications with lower risk for breastfeeding mothers.

- Administer medications immediately after a breastfeeding session to minimise the infant's exposure.

- Avoid prescribing long-acting medications that could lead to higher drug concentrations in breast milk.

- Infants on breastfeeding should for any signs of adverse effects related to the prescribed medication (Table E.1).

- Provide clear instructions to the mother about any precautions or signs that may indicate the infant is experiencing adverse effects.

- Avoid prescribing multiple medications that could lead to additive effects in the infant.

- Discuss the risks and benefits of any proposed treatment and involve the patient in the decision-making process.

- Additionally, consider consulting with specialists in perinatal medicine, obstetrics or paediatrics for complex cases.

Clinical Dental Pharmacology, First Edition. Edited by Kamran Ali.
© 2024 John Wiley & Sons Ltd. Published 2024 by John Wiley & Sons Ltd.

Table E.1 Drug Prescription to Breastfeeding Mothers

Category	Avoid	Suitable alternatives
Analgesics	NSAIDs, e.g., aspirin or ibuprofen in high doses	Paracetamol Codeine
Antimicrobials	Tetracyclines (risk of tooth discolouration), Metronidazole, Fluconazole, Itraconazole	Penicillins, e.g., amoxicillin Cephalosporins Macrolides, e.g., azithromycin Clindamycin, Topical Nystatin, Topical Miconazole
Local anaesthetics	Articaine	Lidocaine

Drug Prescriptions in Patients with Hepatic Disease

Prescribing drugs to patients with established liver disease requires careful consideration due to compromised metabolism of drugs in the liver. Here are some general guidelines to follow:

- Consult with the patient's medical physician and hepatologist to gain advice regarding the status of patient's liver health, recent liver function tests and advice regarding drug prescriptions.

- Consider reducing the dose of drugs (usually to half) to avoid undesirable side effects, especially for medications know to be hepatoxic (Table F.1).

- Keep a vigilant watch for signs of hepatotoxicity, including jaundice, elevated liver enzymes, and changes in mental status and liver function tests in consultation with patient's medical physician.

- Advise against alcohol consumption.

- Educate patients about the importance of adhering to prescribed medications and promptly reporting any signs of adverse effects.

Clinical Dental Pharmacology, First Edition. Edited by Kamran Ali.
© 2024 John Wiley & Sons Ltd. Published 2024 by John Wiley & Sons Ltd.

Table F.1 Drug Prescription in Patients with Hepatic Disease

Category	Avoid	Alternatives
Analgesics	Non-steroidal anti-inflammatory drugs Opioids	Paracetamol in low dose
Antibiotics	Metronidazole Azithromycin Clindamycin Azole antifungals	Penicillins, e.g., amoxicillin Tetracycline Nystatin
Local anaesthetics	Lidocaine	Articaine
Others	Diazepam Midazolam Flumazenil Carbamazepine Phenytoin	Lorazepam

APPENDIX G

Drug Prescriptions in Patients with Renal Disease

Prescribing drugs to patients with chronic kidney disease (CKD) requires careful consideration due to compromised renal excretion of drugs. Here are some general guidelines to follow:

- Consult with the patient's medical physician and nephrologist to gain advice regarding the status of patient's liver health, recent renal function tests and advice regarding drug prescriptions.

- Avoid drugs with known risk of nephrotoxicity, e.g., aminoglycosides and NSAIDs (Table G.1).

- Consider reducing the dose of drugs (usually to half) to avoid undesirable side effects, especially for medications know to be nephrotoxic.

- Consult with the patient's medical physician to identify signs of nephrotoxicity, including changes in urine output, serum creatinine levels, electrolyte imbalance.

- Educate patients about the importance of adhering to prescribed medications and promptly reporting any signs of adverse effects.

Clinical Dental Pharmacology, First Edition. Edited by Kamran Ali.
© 2024 John Wiley & Sons Ltd. Published 2024 by John Wiley & Sons Ltd.

Table G.1 Drug Prescription in Patients with Renal Disease

Category	Avoid	Alternatives
Analgesics	NSAIDS, e.g., aspirin Tramadol	Paracetamol Codeine
Antimicrobials	Aminoglycosides Cephalexin Tetracycline Fluconazole Itraconazole Acyclovir Valaciclovir	Penicillin V Amoxicillin Azithromycin Clindamycin Metronidazole
Local anaesthetics		Lidocaine Articaine
Others	Carbamazepine Gabapentin	Midazolam Flumazenil

Index

Note: *Italicized* and **bold** page numbers refer to figures and tables, respectively

Clinical Dental Pharmacology, First Edition. Edited by Kamran Ali.
© 2024 John Wiley & Sons Ltd. Published 2024 by John Wiley & Sons Ltd.